"It does not re........ .... Science, Exercise Physiology, or Health Sciences to live a healthy life and stay physically fit. The information provided within this book gives you a solid foundation as to how your body works and what it takes to maintain it in optimal health. By simply utilizing this basic information in conjunction with some discipline and determination, you can achieve and maintain your lifestyle change for now and forever! I know this because I live it, I teach it, and it has become my passion to educate the world; re-gifting the gift of life!"

–Joe Carson, BS/CPT

YOUR BODY
YOUR LIFE
YOURSELF

YOUR BODY
YOUR LIFE
YOURSELF
KNOWLEDGE IS POWER

TATE PUBLISHING & *Enterprises*

• JOE CARSON

Published by Tate Publishing & Enterprises, LLC
127 E. Trade Center Terrace | Mustang, Oklahoma 73064 USA
1.888.361.9473 | www.tatepublishing.com

Tate Publishing is committed to excellence in the publishing industry. The company reflects the philosophy established by the founders, based on Psalm 68:11,
"The Lord gave the word and great was the company of those who published it."

Book design copyright © 2009 by Tate Publishing, LLC. All rights reserved.
Cover design by Janae J. Glass
Interior design by Nathan Harmony

Published in the United States of America

ISBN: 978-1-60696-497-2
1. Health & Fitness: Weight Loss
2. Health & Fitness: Healthy Living
08.12.11

TABLE OF CONTENTS

INTRODUCTION

Many in modern society have found themselves in a much too common place of living for the day, putting their fitness and health as a distant priority. I am all too familiar with this cycle, as it consumed me for a number of years and left me at a peak weight of 354 pounds.

I reached a startling realization one evening as I saw my reflection in the mirror and had a heart-to-heart with myself. The truth was that there was no *easy* way out and nobody could do it for me.

With this, my journey to lose the weight began with a vengeance, as I sought any and every way possible to shed the pounds. Just like everyone else in the world who has decided to take this plunge, I wanted the results immediately if not sooner.

I researched all of the popular weight-loss programs (point counters, meal delivery services, etc.) and diets out there, quickly discovering that they are not in the business of effective weight loss or health at all; they are in the business of making mega-million-dollar profits by playing on the emotions of those seeking weight loss and better health.

The "results" in a bottle was next. Just like everyone else, I wanted the easiest/fastest way to make the pounds disappear. Everyone knows that exercise is hard work, and it is really hard work for someone who is morbidly obese. The more I looked at these "miracles in a bottle," the more I discovered that not only do these things not work for long-term results, they are down right dangerous!

Now with two of the "quick and simple" avenues considered and ruled out, this really narrows my options for a fast/easy avenue to lose the weight. There is just one more to examine, bariatric surgery (stomach stapling, stomach bands, gastric bypass, etc). These surgeries are becoming more popular and are showing some success for what they do, but that is only one side of the coin.

There are too many of these surgeries being performed on people who are not appropriate candidates, thusly creating an enormous influx of profit potential for cosmetic/bariatric surgeons because this method is viewed as "a quick fix" yet creating permanent and often fatal consequences for their patients unnecessarily.

The complications associated with bariatric surgery include but are not limited to: infection, malnutrition, increased sensitivity to certain foods, malabsorption of nutrients (attributed to the lack of digestion in the stomach), and in some cases *death*!

The truth is, there is no quick fix/easy way to approach a healthy weight loss that is sustainable. This way of thinking totally misses the mark for attaining health, body composition, and fitness goals then sustaining them permanently. The easy diet, magic pill, miracle surgeries just do not exist in a practical world.

If all of the hyped-up programs were effective, the American population would not be in an outrageous state of poor health, which can be attributed to obesity and poor lifestyle habits. However, what does exist is the information contained within this book to help you formulate a no-fail approach that will not only help you to lose the weight just as I did but also join me in keeping it off *forever*! The coolest thing about this approach is once you have adopted the basic principals permanently in your life, everything becomes second nature to you and then the rest is virtually effortless!

Now which is better? A permanent, cost-effective, and healthy means to weight loss and improved health that is designed by a health and fitness professional who has been there, done that, or becoming another victim of good marketing and emotional manipulation by a large corporation who has no practical foundation to be offering anything for weight loss or health improvement? With the "trending" companies, you are destined to fail and suffer potentially life-altering (if not life-ending) consequences along the way, all the while unnecessarily expending precious resources that can be better utilized for something with benefit. This stuff does not work; if it did, America would not be the most unhealthy and most obese nation in the world!

I chose door number one, and it works!

The "your body, your life, yourself" approach is a matter of empowerment through integrity, education, and adopting a sustainable lifestyle change that will facilitate permanent weight loss, increase energy levels, decrease potential for serious health problems related to obesity, and give you a permanent zeal for a prolonged quality and quantity of life.

It is now time to sit back and enjoy a good book that will give you the information and encouragement necessary to change your life forever—for the better!

Welcome to *Your Body, Your Life, Yourself!*

ABOUT THE AUTHOR

JOSEPH G. CARSON, BS/CPT

I currently hold two Bachelors of Science degrees, two nationally recognized personal training certifications (NASM, and SCW), a certified fitness professional certification (APEX), and a Sports Nutrition Specialist certification (SCW). I am also master trainer and owner of Success Fitness Personal Training Services in Tulsa, Oklahoma, and have performed over 10,000 session hours professionally.

After having experienced a natural weight loss of 177 pounds in fifteen months, I have not only maintained my success but now help others professionally to experience the same level of results that I have enjoyed for over nine years.

I consider myself an extremely passionate trainer and have discovered that by building my clients from the inside out, I can help them to emotionally embrace the challenges associated with making lifestyle changes and ensure permanent success.

This book is dedicated to Jesus Christ my Lord and Savior. Also to my beautiful wife, who has given me the love and support necessary to give each and every client 110 percent session after session, and to my clients who inspire me daily to be the very best trainer and role model possible.

The purpose of this book is simple. I want for those who have experienced the same struggles that I have with weight and health to finally have a realistic tool that is designed with just one goal in mind—your permanent success!

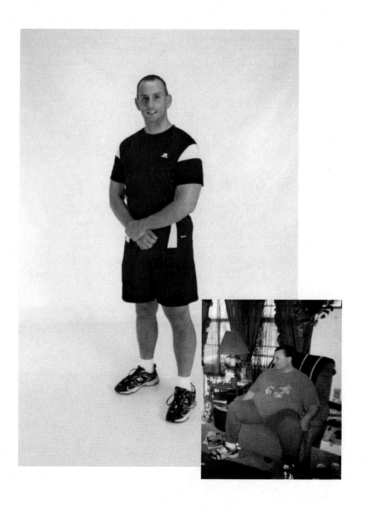

THIS IS THE STORY

Just how did I manage to lose 177 pounds in just fifteen months completely naturally and without any surgery? We will address this but will more importantly address how I got to the state where I had 177 pounds to lose and the realization that it took for me to make the changes. This is the basic story of where I started and how I came to be a renowned health and fitness expert.

I am sharing this story with you because we all have to start somewhere, and understanding just exactly what it took for me and the motivations behind this massive undertaking may give you the extra bit of encouragement and knowledge that it takes to identify key components in your life that may help you to be successful on the same journey without succumbing to the many pitfalls that can cause major setbacks.

All through my childhood and high school I had always been able to easily maintain a healthy weight, as well as staying active in sports and boyhood activities. I enlisted in the United States Marine Corps at seventeen, easily passing the military physical fitness testing and service requirements. This takes away my excuse of saying that I had been a chubby kid all of my life as a means of justification for letting myself go.

In my early twenties I hit a steel reinforced brick wall in my life, and everything that I knew as "security and safety" were all gone. This left me in the most emotionally volatile period I had ever experienced. By this time I had gotten out of the Marines and had no real standards to adhere to for weight or fitness, so I decided that I was going to turn to my love of food for comfort and security.

My new motto was, "I do not have anyone to impress, so I'm going to eat what I want, when I want, and as much as I want." Boy did I ever pay for this way of thinking. I began to quickly pack on the pounds, as I was eating purely for the joy and satisfaction of it.

I did not go to the "super-mega buffet," pull up a chair to the line, and just throw down every day. However, I did not hesitate to get my money's worth. When eating for satisfaction, you will discover that it's the foods that are the worst for you that make you feel the best (well, at the time).

The trouble is this "food high" does not last, and before long it becomes a terrible "food low." When I began noticing that I could not keep clothes in my closet that actually fit and that none of the major department stores carried stylish clothes in my size, I began to pick up on the fact that I had a problem.

I also noticed that my social life dynamics had changed quite a bit in all areas from work, friends, the band I played in, the way I was treated by strangers, and the way that I felt.

I no longer looked at myself as a strong, confident, and attractive person. Rather, what I saw looking back at me in the mirror totally disgusted me. I was a 354-pound example of misery and self-loathing, not who I really was or wanted to be.

One evening after a shower, I got out of the stall and noticed my reflection in the full-length shower door mirror. I was standing there in all of my glory thinking to myself, *Your butt looks like a wad of chewed bubble gum; you need to do something about that.* It was at this point that I had the reality check that nobody could make this change for me and that either I wanted it or I didn't; there was no in between.

I also had just found out that I was going to be a father for the first time and took the iron skillet of reality to the face that I was going to have to step up and lead by example for this child. My life was no longer just about me.

This turn of events made me realize the time had come to turn my way of thinking (and feeling sorry for myself) around and call on my inner strength to seek resources to start making things happen.

Being in college at the time really worked out well, as I was able to take advantage of several human nutrition, physiology, and health-sciences classes to begin my academic journey toward losing the weight and getting my life back on track. I used these classes in addition to resources that I found on the Internet and library to stuff my brain with as much relevant information as possible to create a highly effective, efficient, sustainable, and safe program.

Just like anyone else, I wanted the weight to come off yesterday and began researching every "quick-fix" option to begin shedding the pounds. What I found out not only alarmed me; it quite honestly ticked me off! There is a multibilliondollar industry in modern American society which focuses on just one thing, playing on the emotions of those who are overweight and unhealthy for the sake of pure profit, not with the true intentions of making a real difference in the lives of consumers.

Consider, if these companies created products/plans that actually worked, we would be among the healthiest countries in the world and have diminishing healthcare costs. Rather, because this industry feeds on greed and mega-profit potential without creating any *real* solutions, we now have the title of the fattest country with some of the highest medical costs in the entire modern world!

Straight up, the commercial junk does not work; there is no quick fix. No miracle diet, no magic pills, no infomercial solution, and no cure-all weight-loss option that is fast, easy, and permanently effective. It just does not exist as a true reality for anything that is sustainable in promoting weight loss and good health.

For me it came down to one basic principal: education combined with sweat equity. This also will apply to you as well. Think about this, how much value do you truly place in something that is easily attainable, other than the fact that it was easy? With this process you will get out of it what you put into it; that is it, no smoke and mirrors, just facts!

Because I had established good groundwork in college, I built upon my basic knowledge by learning about the specific nutritional requirements of each of the body's functions/processes; then I researched which foods were the most nutrient dense without unnecessary/empty calories.

By combining good quality foods in a competently designed nutrition program and a solid determination to refuse to deviate, I began to shed the pounds right away. Once this process was in place, I researched exercise and activities that efficiently burn calories and provide the most weight-loss and fitness benefits.

This combination worked out to be an extraordinary amount of cardio respiratory training (seventy-five minutes per day) combined with high-intensity strength/circuit training, and a strict regimen of activities (bike riding, tennis, etc.) outside of the gym. This is the hardcore plan that had me losing between seven to eleven pounds per week.

Understand that I was in the gym for two hours per day, six days per week, and when I was not in the gym, I was active doing something.

I must admit that in the onset, I thought that this was going to be miserably laborious and was going to leave me tired all of the time. Much to my surprise, I was more energetic and felt better than I had in years! It also was quite an emotional victory to hop onto the scale once per week and see the numbers just dropping like rocks. There are few things that feed your motivational fire more than the logs of success!

For many, the chances of actually going to this extreme in the onset are going to be slim and would most likely be counterproductive. However, if you closely examine the steps that I took and begin implementing them into your life at levels that are sustainable, you will see that what you have to gain are: knowledge, empowerment, and dedication, all the while watching the pounds disappear forever!

I determined my final weight by simply dividing my heaviest weight of 354 pounds directly in half and deciding that this was going to be my goal. How many people can say that they have lost an entire person? Because this fit within normal, good health standards for my body, I managed to safely reach this weight of 177 pounds and maintain it.

As a guy with a new body, I wanted to make the most of it, so I began focused strength training to add muscle mass and definition to my somewhat saggy (but still slimmer and healthier!) body. With several years of diligence and hard training, I have managed to put twenty pounds of muscle onto my body and build upon my good health.

Through the course of the weight loss, I had a number of people I worked with that were just amazed at such a radical transformation taking place before their eyes. So obviously, many were inquiring as to what it was that I was doing, and before long I was coaching several of them, teaching the things that I had learned that were working for me.

Eventually this coaching turned into training, and after some soul searching within my career path, I decided that helping people discover the true zeal of life through health and fitness is exactly what my calling in this world is. I became a Certified Personal Trainer, and got a job in a health club as the Fitness Manager.

I now have moved out of the commercial health club environment and into my own private studio, where I spend my days helping people just like me and you to live healthier, happier, and longer lives.

Hopefully you enjoyed this summarized version of my lifestyle change story and how my hard work, dedication, and passion can now be put to good use by helping you to begin your journey of *Your body, Your life, Yourself.*

WEIGHT LOSS DEFINED

For most, weight loss is an abstract concept that normally centers on one's outward appearance. Determining just exactly how to go about losing weight and developing an understanding of how best to keep the weight off is an ever-growing task with all of the creative marketing and hype surrounding this ever-growing, multi-billion dollar industry.

Why are we fat? Just exactly how and why does that happen? Fat storage is a primal survival mechanism that is ancestral in nature and can be traced back for centuries as a way of coping with periods of famine. Even though the dynamics of our everyday lives have radically evolved, why is it that our fat storage mechanisms have not?

There are many reasons for weight gain and obesity, taking the factors of genetic makeup, hormonal imbalances, physiological maladies, poor-quality food, and sedentary lifestyle into consideration. There is more to it than "energy in, energy out," and this understanding is the primary key to unlocking your success in weight loss.

Which of the above factors apply to you and your lifestyle? Understand that regardless of whatever your primary contributor to weight gain is, it can be overcome and you can reach a healthy weight/body composition. The word *can't* does not factor into the weight-loss equation at any juncture. Self-defeating phrases like "I can't lose weight because my whole family is big," and "I'm just built like that" facilitate justified failure. There may be genetic factors that are a contributor; however, they do not have to have prevalence. It may take an extra cardio session every week, spotless nutritional habits, and a bit more diligence, but you can achieve your goals, and they will be well rewarded as you age, guaranteed!

The traditional approach is to find out what the latest diet is and get on it, hoping for the best but not really knowing the facts or consequences. Please know that the word *diet* in this context is another word for structured failure. There is no specific "diet" (in the traditional sense) that you are going to be able to get on, lose the weight, and then sustain that diet forever in order to keep the weight off. Rather you must adopt a lifestyle change process in order to facilitate proper weight loss and sustainability.

Also, please understand that trying to lose weight without proper exercise is very much discouraged. I know that there are just tons of the latest programs and plans on the market that promise these awesome results without you having to get off of your couch.

Now, think about that for a moment. Does this really make any sense at all? The human body is designed to be active and to work hard; that is just the way it is. Do you really think that a plan that encourages you to be sedentary would really be healthy or beneficial to you or your long-term health? If the entire process were just effortless and completely easy, do you think you would see enough value in what you had accomplished to make the necessary sacrifices and changes to maintain it? Of course not.

It is at this point when the reality check must take place and you develop the understanding that just like with any-thing else in life that is worth doing, weight loss and fitness is a process in which you are going to get out of it what you put into it. A maximal effort (in conjunction with information in this book) will always yield a maximal result, whereas a mediocre effort will always yield a mediocre (at best) result.

Now let's develop a basic understanding of body com-position and define what type of weight you want to be los-ing. The concept a pound, is a pound, is a pound does not apply to body composition. Your body-weight is made up of four basic components: lean mass (muscle and organ tissue), water (up to 70 percent), bone, and fat. Now, in looking at these four basic components, which ones would we want to see less of on your body for the sake of good health?

Lean mass, specifically muscle, is metabolic tissue and aids in elevating your metabolic rate (the rate at which you burn calories for ready energy); strong muscles also lead to strong connective tissues (ligaments and tendons), strong bones, and facilitate daily tasks. So, you will want to add and maintain as much of this body-weight component as possible.

Bone and the mineral density composing the bones in your skeletal system are extremely important to have as strong as possible in order to ensure structural integrity and injury prevention. So, you do not want to be losing anything there.

Water-weight—now here is an interesting component. Water, though vital to good health and normal body function, can also be stored in excess amounts within fat cells as a result of poor nutritional and hydration habits. So, losing some water-weight through the course of the weight-loss process is normal and not always a bad thing. However, it is still not your primary goal.

Fat—this is the guy that you want to focus on losing the most of. All of the above body components are good for you and are imperative to your good health. There are two kinds of fat in the human body: visceral (abdominal and around the organs) and subcutaneous (adipose tissue beneath the skin) fats. These guys are what your primary focus for eradication should be. Fat is stored lipids in your adipose tissue (tissue that contains fat storage cells) as a reserve *energy* resource. This is a means of your body trying to protect itself from famine or a time of insufficient energy necessary for life function.

Fat as a whole in healthy levels is a good thing because it does do what its primary focus is, and that is to provide reserve energy, but it also insulates the body from temperature extremes and provides cushioning for the musculoskeletal system and organ cavity.

Think about this and the key word here; *energy*. Just as with any other energy source (electricity, fossil fuels, etc.) you must utilize the resource in order to deplete it. Fat is no different. You must utilize this surplus resource in the way of exercise and activity, while not replenishing what you are displacing through proper nutrition.

For example, this is a lot like a battery in your car. If you unhook the charging system and operate the car's electrical system solely on the battery, sooner or later it will run dead, and you will have depleted its energy resources because they are not being replenished by the charging system.

This is the obvious and correct approach to healthy weight loss. There are no "super-miracle tuna and green tea diets," "easy mega fat-burner pills," or other infomercial gimmicks that are permanently effective in helping you lose weight. Unfortunately their goal is to just make your wallet slimmer, not your waist line

This is the "secret" that the weight loss industry does not want you to know. By learning just exactly how your body utilizes the foods you eat for energy, understanding how/why to exercise (primary fat-loss catalyst), eradicating bad habits, and adopting a healthy way of living, your permanent results are assured!

"A healthy body is always a beautiful body, but a beautiful body is not always a healthy body." Keep this thought close to your heart and understand that you are working toward a healthier body and way of living; losing fat, inches, and body-weight are all exciting by-products of this permanent process.

MOTIVATION

Initially for me, losing weight was a matter of obligation and emotional dissatisfaction, as I just had a new little person come into my world that permanently changed my life dynamics and priorities. I was forced to ask myself, "How am I going to take care of and provide for this child if I am not even taking care of myself? Am I living the right life to show her by example how she should grow up and live?"

Often we do not take the time in our busy daily lives to contemplate the future for ourselves or our loved ones and what adverse effects our neglected health can have on them. I did not want to fall into this category, because I thought it selfish to compromise the potential quality of my child's life due to my lack of motivation.

This is a very serious gut check and leads many of us to further evaluate what is really important in our lives and leads us to ask ourselves, how do we want our quality of life in the future to be? The truth is family and social dynamics do not leave us by ourselves through the course of life; we have direct and indirect influence on the lives of each and every person around us. How we conduct ourselves and care for ourselves has an impact (often adverse) on other people besides us.

With this, we need to establish a means and method of determining just exactly what your motivation to lose weight and adopt a lifestyle change is and where it comes from.

For many (myself included), the cosmetic/aesthetic appeal initiated the primary impact and made me realize just how bad of shape I was really in. In my professional experience, I have had few weight-loss clients come to me with the first thing that they mention being improved health, quality of life, and longevity. Initially they ask, "Can you make this fat right here go away? I hate the way that this looks!" At this time I then need to make the determination of what their true source of motivation is and if it is just superficial or if it runs deeper.

Cosmetic appeal is just an actual by-product of the weight-loss process. Though it's difficult to not focus solely on aesthetic appeal, you must always know and understand that good health, wellness, and fitness are always a primary goal.

A famous tagline at my gym is, "A beautiful body is not always a healthy body, but a healthy body is always a beautiful body!" This means that if you will simply maintain a focus on the health-improving benefits of your new way of life, you will soon see that your body will begin the transformation into its full cosmetic potential.

What are the dynamics in your life that have led you to seek out a solution for weight loss? On a piece of paper, make a list of the top ten reasons that you want to lose weight. Then once this list is made, organize it by priority, with one being the most important.

Now that you have your top ten list, write out beside each

item whether it is driven by an ideal (i.e. my new jeans make me look fat), perception (how you or others see you), peer (friends or family included), or emotion (sadness, happiness, depression, anxiety, etc.). Be honest with yourself and understand that nobody else has to see this list other than you.

Let's examine this list now and see where these items originate. You now want to create a second list, this time only listing the items that have only "emotion" next to them. These are the items in which you will see the most personal value through the course of this process. All of the others are superficial in nature and will not give you any substance to call on for strength or determination when faced with challenge.

Here is an example of how your list might look:

Top Ten List Why I Want to Lose Weight

1. My wife does not find me attractive anymore. (peer)
2. I have no energy to do things that I like, and I hate it! (emotion)
3. Making friends is tough; people just do not like those who are fat. (perception)
4. None of my clothes fit anymore. (ideal)
5. I have a great family, and I need to be healthy to take care of them. (emotion)
6. I always get passed up for promotions at work, and it's because I'm fat. (perception)
7. I feel as though I'm letting myself go and food is my only comfort. (emotion)
8. My sister says the floor shakes when I walk past her. (peer)

9. I went to the doctor, and he told me that I'm at high risk for diabetes and heart attack. (peer)
10. I do not want to have to be buried in a special casket and people to make fun of me at my funeral. (emotion)

My List That Matters
1. I have a great family, and I need to be healthy to take care of them. (emotion)
2. I do not want to have to be buried in a special casket and people to make fun of me at my funeral. (emotion)
3. I have no energy to do things that I like, and I hate it! (emotion)
4. I feel as though I'm letting myself go and food is my only comfort. (emotion)

This is now your sheet of reflection that you will use through the entirety of the process and will help to keep you emotionally on track when all else seems to fail. Though many of the things around us have an effect on how we feel, those are simply feelings of someone else being imposed on us, rather than your feelings and will not have as much significance to you as what you feel for yourself.

We have now established a solid foundation as to why you want to lose the weight, and as you have discovered through this simple exercise, the real reasoning goes far deeper than the tight clothes or the social implications.

Human beings are emotional creatures; a majority of our decisions and thought processes originate from our emotions and how we feel. Because of this, it is important to realize that when making significant changes to your lifestyle, it is important to harness that emotional energy to feed your determination and get you through the challenging times. The sense of accomplishment from conquering adversities will just feed your desire to persevere further.

Now the next step is to understand that there are no magic diets, no miracle pills, no weight loss in a box, and the truth is there is no *easy* way to do it correctly. However, this does not mean that the process has to be intolerable or unattainable; we just need to establish some basic groundwork to build upon.

With this, understand that nobody can do this for you, and you cannot do it for anybody other than yourself. Meaning, do not try to lose weight for any reason other than those that are deeply embedded within your own heart, because through every true challenge you face, your strength to persevere will always come from your heart, not your muscles.

You will learn how to set realistic goals that will help you to achieve milestones and keep you emotionally on track. Often, the misconception exists that we can "get back" to the weight or the way we looked when we were younger, and unfortunately this goal is not always appropriate or realistic. Our bodies change through the course of time, and with that so does the mean (healthy maintenance) composition (age, gender, height, weight, and body-fat percentage) ratio.

Many find themselves setting these unrealistic goals when pursuing a weight loss (diet) program and often lose motivation and fail because their goals and methods have no scientific or practical basis. With this, do not rely on any data (body-weight, body-fat percentage, etc.) that you see on any of the commercial weight-loss Web sites or in any of the magazines as being the right numbers for you.

The most reliable means for determining what your ideal body weight/composition is to inquire with your physician when you go in for your pre-process physical. Please understand that each and every person on the planet is different and there are no "across the board" standards that are relevant to every individual and body type.

Now you must take one final and crucial step in the motivational process—*get excited*! By the time you finish this book and place all of the processes into practice, you will be empowered to charge forward and never look back, becoming a success story rather than just another failure statistic.

GETTING DOWN TO THE BASICS

There is only one tried, true, and proven method to effective and sustainable weight loss. This is through education and learning how to eat, exercise, and live an active/healthy lifestyle. You must develop an understanding that even though calorie intake is important, it is not the sole way to weight loss and good health.

In order for you to be completely successful, you will have to learn a system of balance in your life and understand that to weigh heavy in any particular thing or area will cause a counterproductive effect and possibly throw you off of your focus.

The expectation is not for you to totally give up foods you like and to live two hours per day on a Stairmaster. However, what you will learn to expect from yourself is developing that sense of synergy between nutrition, exercise, activity, and your healthy lifestyle.

This means that you should not feel like a slug for having a slice of pie or a cookie once in a while (in extreme moderation), but this also means that you do not want to have an entire plate of "bad" food, then follow it up with one of each dessert you see to satisfy a craving. The truth is, by eating like this, you will not only feel bad physically (especially if you have been eating healthy awhile), but you will also feel bad emotionally for having "fallen off of the wagon."

Life is short, and you should make the most of it and enjoy yourself, all the while preserving your quality of life in longevity. What I want to teach you within this book is the information necessary for you to make informed decisions about how to get healthy and stay that way.

Though it may seem laborious and arduous in the interim, the exercise component of your lifestyle change is going to become your best friend, not only through the weight-loss process, but also through the rest of your happy, healthy life.

Just as with finding balance in nutrition, you do not have to set up a cot in the locker room of your local gym and take up housekeeping in order to lose weight and be healthy. However, I will tell you that the exercise is not just important to your success, it is vital!

I could go into pages upon pages of science to solidify my point, but that is not what this book is about. What I want to communicate to you is just a very simple, straightforward, and structured approach on how you should exercise safely and effectively to not only lose weight but to increase energy levels, elevate metabolism, build bone mineral density, increase strength, strengthen and stabilize joints, and stimulate good cardiovascular health, just to name a few of the benefits.

All of this while lowering your chances of suffering from type 2 diabetes, diminishing risk for heart attack, lowering potential for hypertension, cutting the chances of osteoporosis and osteoarthritis, reversing the effects of aging, increasing energy levels, reducing body fat percentages, diminishing aches and pains, improving digestion, improving quality of sleep/rest, improving love life, and the list continues !

It is true that you can exercise too much and make for a counter-productive condition; this is typical of those who become obsessive and do not have the education to know any better. What you are looking for in this area again is just knowing how to make educated choices in order to maintain balance. Typically one hour of intense/focused exercise per day is plenty sufficient to help you reach your goals.

I will be the first to admit that I was borderline obsessive and was in the gym for two hours per day, six days per week in order to achieve the level of weight loss that I had in such a short time frame. The primary difference is that I had educated myself and was utilizing a very structured approach to manipulate my metabolic rate and utilize fat calories for energy.

This technique is very precise and, to be honest with you, was really tough to do during the process. There is absolutely nothing fun or enjoyable about having to go that hardcore for that long in the beginning. I do not recommend this approach to you and would discourage anyone who does not have the information or the emotional drive from ever attempting such a daunting feat. It is always better to have the process take a little longer and be successful than to try to hurry through it and set yourself up for failure.

Discovering the harmonic balance and synergy within all of the components of your life (nutrition, exercise, activity, work, family, and recreation) is extremely important and is among the most crucial of changes to be made in your life-style change process.

For many, organization is the key challenge in maintaining a sense of balance. The best approach to introducing structured organization into your life is to analyze each aspect one item at a time, developing a system that works for you, rather than trying to master the whole project (or group of projects) at once. These organizational skills will help you later in the process as you *make* (key word here!) time to exercise, to prepare your meals, and to find recreational activities that are good for mind and body.

Knowing your current state of health is also going to be crucial to the success and safety of your lifestyle change process. How long has it been since you have had a thorough physical examination by your physician? For many that can be way too long! This step is a must before beginning any fitness or nutrition program (this one included). Visit with your doctor and have a complete, thorough physical.

This information and guidance could potentially save your life, as you may have medical issues with little or no immediate symptoms that you would not know about otherwise, or a condition that requires a specific approach through nutrition and/or exercise.

Be sure to take your data sheets and plan of action (all you will create further along in this book) for your doctor's review, to discuss your findings and goals with him/her. Inquire about ideal weight/body composition for yourself as well. You may also quickly discover that you will receive another positive avenue of support and guidance to further you toward your goals, because many physicians are strong advocates of healthy lifestyle adjustments.

There are a few little things that many of us tend to forget through the course of a day that can make or break our overall success. One of these is our commitment to ourselves as an initial priority, rather than a secondary afterthought.

So many in modern society have a "could have, would have, and should have, but didn't" mentality as it relates to caring for their physical, emotional, and psychological health. All of these components play into our overall wellness and longevity and could lead us down a path of infinite successes or doomed for continual disaster.

A simplified way to look at your long-term health is this: how your body treats you as you age is contingent upon how you are treating it now. Simply put, if you are not eating healthy, exercising regularly, managing stress, and keeping clean and active lifestyle habits, it's not a matter of if, but when and how badly you will pay for it, often with prematurely fatal or debilitating consequences.

Think about this for a second. If you are not proactively caring for your body and your health, you are harming yourself. Why would anyone in their right mind ever consciously decide that they would like to suffer a slow, painful, miserable, and premature death simply because they were too lazy to do anything about it when they could? Does not make sense, does it? Why would anybody do that?

It is much easier (and more enjoyable long term) to live proactively and know that if you do not take care of yourself, it's not a matter of if but when and how badly you're going to pay for it than it is to suffer the horrific consequences alternatively (this includes smoking and alcohol use as well!).

Health insurance is on an eternal climb; instances of heart disease, type 2 diabetes, hypertension, and countless other conditions of concern are on the radical increase with the only end in sight coming from a significant shift in how we currently live in our convenience-based lifestyle, adopting a new way of thinking.

Sounds like a lot of gloom and doom speak, and as a matter of fact, it is! I wish that I could tell you that America was not the fattest nation in the world. I would do anything to be able to say that all Americans have embraced as a whole the value in a healthy lifestyle and have made it a priority; and I would sell the farm to be able to say that our health-care system was responsible for providing the educational components to initiate a proactive response to all of the above, but that is just not the case.

However, what you are reading is the beginning of a movement that starts with your success and learning to lead as an example for others. By you becoming a champion for the sake of health, fitness, and wellness through your change in lifestyle, you will have the life-improving opportunity to reach friends, family, coworkers, peers, and those around you to share the blessing that is living healthy and happy on through your golden years.

The whole purpose of this book and this program is to empower everyone who wants and or needs to make changes in their lifestyle to facilitate better long- and short-term health with the unadulterated information necessary to do just that successfully and without a bunch of commercial nonsense (which incidentally is only guaranteed to make your pocket book slimmer!).

The previous chapters have set the groundwork for establishing motivation and for understanding the basics. We have also established some key concepts that will help to change the way you look at this program as opposed to other diets and commercial "gimmicks" on the market.

If you have never kept any kind of diary or journal before, here is your chance to learn to keep possibly the most important records of your life. I know that with the busy day-to-day hustle and a thousand other things to do on a daily basis, keeping a journal may seem like another arduous task that you'd rather do without; but please understand that not only does this record keep you on track, but it will help with accountability.

There are a number of commercially printed journal books available that you can use for keeping these records. Also, I have included a basic journal in the back of this book to give you a head start and give you some examples of what your records should look like.

You do not have to keep this journaling process up forever, but once you master the crucial concepts, you will quickly understand how helpful it is to know where you began and what your progress is on a daily basis, as well as the educational/accountability data contained within.

The following chapters will take you into the actual processes necessary to begin Your body, Your life, Yourself!

FOOD: GAS, DIESEL, OR ROCKET FUEL!

"Over the lips, through the gums, look out, stomach, here it comes," is a traditional approach to nutrition for many. For others, nutrition is a matter of picking up whatever is convenient to satisfy hunger pangs while on the go. Let's face it, food in common society is plentiful, and boy does a lot of it taste good! These components in part are not necessarily bad; but pair them up with a very busy and convenience-based modern way of thinking/living, and it can (and has) created a recipe for disaster.

This chapter will give you a strong foundation as to how best to approach nutrition and develop an understanding of why you eat, how your body utilizes food for energy, what happens if you consume too much/too little food or eat the wrong foods, and what foods are healthy for you.

Once you have a handle on nutritional basics, you will quickly discover that the real secret to losing weight and keeping it off does not lie in your ability to count calories or trying to adhere to the latest and greatest "magic tea and tuna diet." Rather, you will see that just by making healthy choices in balanced portions, you will instantly feel better and begin to even see the difference.

It's kind of funny to think about it in these terms, but many people feel as if they are being deprived if they do not get to eat what they want and as much as they want. Actually they are most deprived because they did eat what they wanted and as much as they wanted. This kind of eating leads to operating in a far greater diminished capacity physically, mentally, and emotionally than they were prior to the monstrous meal, due to their body being in a state of digestive resource distress (digestion always gets first energy resource).

Time has come to examine priorities and what genuinely satisfies each of us.

With this said, there is a lot of exciting information within this chapter, which barely scratches the surface as it relates to nutritional science. The point is just to give you a simplified approach that will immediately empower you to make educated and conscious decisions about what you eat.

Nutritional supplementation is a common area in which many people find themselves very confused and misinformed. Because it is very relevant, we are going to address this potentially serious issue first.

Please understand that currently, nutritional supplements are not regulated for quality or efficacy and virtually anyone with an encapsulator and sufficient supply of cornstarch can get into the supplement business and promise you the world in a bottle.

With this there are a number of very dangerous stimulant

and herbal-based weight-loss supplements that can not only have adverse side effects while you are taking them, such as nervousness, light headedness, headaches, cramps, rapid heart rate, and sudden fatigue, some of these supplements can cause permanent damage to your liver, heart, neurological system, kidneys, other delicate life systems, and even death!

The marketing is the only good thing about these supplements, as they are not at all beneficial to getting you to your goals and may do permanent or fatal harm in the process. It's just not worth the risk for a short-term benefit (yes, this means that any weight lost with a supplement is non-sustainable and is guaranteed to return and will be much harder to take back off). You will have to make the appropriate changes in your lifestyle and eating habits to sustain any weight loss permanently; this is just fact.

Many people when first making changes to their way of eating and exercising will have a tough time with energy balance, as their bodies are becoming accustomed to the shifts in the amount of energy in versus energy out. This is normal and will quickly rectify itself to the better in a relatively short amount of time with diligence and the aid of a few simple processes.

By taking a good-quality (do not look for discount/bargain brands) multivitamin, you will help to supplement your daily nutritional intake by providing your body with the vitamins and minerals necessary for optimal function and metabolic performance. For many (women especially), deficiencies in iron are becoming problematic due to poor nutritional habits, and it may be necessary to choose a vitamin complex compounded with additional iron to satisfy this deficiency.

A simple blood test at the time of your pre-program physical can tell you if this additional supplementation is necessary.

Because it is extremely difficult to acquire all of these beneficial/essential nutrients (vitamins/minerals) through simple nutrition alone, it is often necessary to supplement them in.

Another nutritional process to address is a "system cleanse." There are a number of products commercially available to aid in this process, and I recommend that you consult with your physician for a recommendation. By taking a digestive system "cleansing" supplement in conjunction with a diet rich in high-fiber foods and sufficient amounts of water, you will prime your digestive system (and your metabolism by association) for optimal function. This will not only facilitate efficient digestion of the much smaller, less complex meals that you will be eating but will also provide you with increased energy levels, improve bathroom regularity, and aid in nutrient uptake.

This process should be done with medical guidance and normally will last the first seven to fourteen days of your lifestyle change process. You may experience more frequent than usual restroom visits during this time, but it does normalize and become more regular once you are off of the "cleansing" product and adapt to the cleaner/healthier way of eating.

There are also studies that suggest that this cleansing and detoxification process has a neurological effect as it relates to leptin levels, which dictate energy storage (glycogen in muscle for immediate energy or fat in adipose tissue for reserve energy, as well as some thyroid function). This is significant, as with increased leptin levels, also comes elevated metabolic rate and working energy capacity.

A cleansing/detoxifying program may look something like this:

Breakfast:
- Fruit smoothie (natural fruit) with protein powder and flax meal, 16 oz. distilled water

Snack:
- 1/4 cup soy nuts, 3 carrot sticks, 1/4 cup grapes, 16 oz. distilled water

Lunch:
- 2 cups fresh baby-spinach salad with broccoli, walnuts, and roasted chicken breast tossed with a vinaigrette dressing made with extra-virgin olive oil, 16 oz. distilled water

Snack:
- 1/4 cup almonds, small apple, 12 oz. distilled water

Dinner:
- 6 oz. baked salmon, 1 cup steamed broccoli, 8 oz. distilled water

This is just a basic idea as to what you should expect when going through this cleansing/detoxifying process. I know that it looks a little daunting, but please understand what you are contrasting and comparing that to and know that by eating in this fashion, you are diminishing distress in your body and creating a prime foundation for a successful weight loss.

Notice that the entirety of the program revolves around simple, clean, fresh foods in modest portions. By eliminating the processed and energy-dense foods from your diet, taking in sufficient dietary fiber, and hydrating well, your body is able to purify and clean out toxic conditions in your digestive tract.

Examining the foods you currently eat will provide you with the information necessary to develop an understanding of how and why your body has stored excess fat as an energy source and how best to approach the modifications process to get your body to utilize these fat stores for energy.

What are your favorite foods? Make a list of your top twenty, then do some research on each one to find out the nutritional data (calories, protein, carbohydrate, fat, saturated fat, and sodium), then take a look at the source of these foods and what the ingredients are (if you can even pronounce many of them).

Pay extra close attention to the nutritional data/information labels on food packages and notice that for many what would be assumed as a single-size portion pack may actually in fact contain multiple portions, and that if you eat the whole package you will need to multiply all of the data (calories, fat, protein, carbohydrate, sugar, sodium, etc.) by the number of servings in that package.

So, for instance, a package of potato chips (small convenience-store bag) says in big writing: 240 calories, 18 grams of fat, 12 grams saturated fat, 28 grams of carbohydrate, and 650 milligrams of sodium. This is bad enough. What is perceived to be one serving (by virtue of its packaging size) is actually 2.25 servings per container (found in small print at the top of the label).

If you consume this entire bag as a single serving, then you have actually consumed 540 calories, 40.5 grams of fat,

27 grams of saturated fat, 63 grams of carbohydrate, and a whopping 1462.5 milligrams of sodium!

Since most potato chips are eaten as an accompaniment to another item (i.e. a sandwich), you can clearly see where this misconception can quickly add up with your daily caloric intake. Beware, there are many (way too many in my opinion) companies that manipulate their data via servings per container to make their product more marketable, as they know most people who look will just notice the "calories" information and not see the multiplier.

Once you have done your homework, be sure that you are sitting down when all of the numbers come together. You will be shocked to see that many of the modern foods consumed on a daily basis have virtually little to no actual (bio-available) nutritional value and are a product of profit maximization efforts rather than solid nutritional development.

Just a simple examination of common, everyday foods will reveal that we are consuming calories on an enormous scale, and the nutritional quality of these calories is minimal. As we go farther along in this chapter, I will explain just what a calorie is, how it works in your body, what are good calories, what calorie sources to avoid, and give you an approach that does not leave you with a calorie counter in hand for every meal.

Have you ever asked yourself, now why would I need to know how many calories are in something I eat? It tastes good, fills the hole, and keeps me from feeling hungry. What does it matter? This is my favorite analogy for answering this common question. Your car's fuel intake system is designed to utilize only a very specific measure of fuel to make the engine run, and the measure changes when the car is at idle or at full speed. Your body works in exactly the same way.

The only difference is your car uses only gasoline, whereas your body uses the food that you put into it for fuel. With your car, you force too much fuel into the engine, it simply chokes down and dies, where in the human body, you force too much fuel into the engine, it simply stores this fuel away (in the form of fat) as a reserve to be used later.

This analogy also applies to the quality of the food that we eat. Consider, you fill up your car with three-quarters of a tank unleaded gasoline but then top it off with a quarter tank of diesel fuel. Sure it will most likely start and will even run; however, it is assured that it will not run well for very long and will perform poorly when placed under demand (sputtering as you hit the gas to get on the expressway).

Because your body has only so many energy resources to allocate to all of the various functions running simultaneously (neurological, muscular, skeletal, digestive, cardiovascular, respiratory, etc.), it sees digestion (its source of renewed energy to run all of these systems) as a top priority and allocates resources accordingly.

However, when you consume an enormous meal with various complex components (even worse with processed foods), your digestive system and your body is placed into a state of distress. This is why you may feel sluggish, tired, and not quite up to par after having consumed a large meal. This is also the time when your body stores surplus energy (fat) the most efficiently, as your metabolic rate becomes compromised.

So, what I'm telling you is this. When you have poor eating habits (too much food, too little food, poor quality food, or any/all of the above) your body is in a state of distress and will always perform in all functions (neurological included) in a diminished capacity. This translates into sub-par performance at work, in activities, information comprehension/retention, exercise performance, and even weight loss.

When your body is in a distressed state, all of its natural self-defense mechanisms are hard at work to protect essential system's integrity (digestion, cardiovascular, respiratory, essential neurological function, etc.). One way that it does this is through the efficient storage of energy resource (fat).

For some there are genetic pitfalls that make fat storage more efficient than for others; and for these types weight loss is most definitely much more of a struggle, but is attainable. I know this because I am one of this unfortunate population that gained up to a maximum weight of 354 pounds by eating popular foods in what I considered satisfying portions. Because of my genetic makeup, I stored a good deal of any/all excess calories as lipids in my adipose tissue (tissue that contains fat storage cells), becoming morbidly obese in a measurably short amount of time.

I have managed to keep my weight off almost nine years to present; however, it is not an easy process. My eating habits are extremely rigid, and my exercise regimen is without compromise. This is to accomplish multiple tasks, the first in maintaining a healthy weight/body composition for good health, but I also must lead by example in my line of work as a health and fitness professional. Simply put, I (as with anyone else having a compromised metabolic state, genetic or other) must remain diligent and determined to stay on track.

The most productive frame of mind for understanding

this extremely complicated concept/process is simplified as, we must eat for the purpose of eating, nothing more, nothing less. Many of us tend to feed our emotions or let cravings dictate our food choices, and both of these causalities can lead to binge eating and extremely efficient weight gain.

Consider and apply this basic empowerment principal in the forefront of your mind as you prepare to consume any food: "Does my body need all of these calories for my current energy needs, or does my brain want this food just because I crave it?" You now can make a conscious decision before you have even consumed the first bite and will know that any excess calories consumed can and often will be stored as reserve energy (fat) even from just one bad meal.

On the flip side of this, understand that eating too little food (a common diet pitfall) is just as bad for you and will hinder your overall results. Too few calories sends your body into starvation mode which invokes primal self defenses, slowing metabolism and promoting a catabolic (breaking down of lean tissue organs included) state for energy. This state also changes brain chemistry and will eventually lead to binge eating and radical fat storage (how many who try this lose lots of weight then gain more than they lost right back).

Now that we know the effects that food has on our body when making poor nutritional choices (I will define this further in this section), we will also now find out what would be considered good nutritional choices and the most optimum way to eat.

I am not a certified nutritionist or dietician, and the purpose of this book is not to put you on any specific nutrition program. However, what we do want to accomplish is communication of some basic information that will empower you to make better choices and nutritional decisions going forward into this lifestyle change process. These are the things that helped me to get a firm foothold on a very complicated and often confusing subject.

How many calories should you be eating through the course of a day? A great way to determine this number is by using the Harris Benedict formula. Do not let the numbers intimidate you. This equation is very simple and will provide you with crucial information as you progress forward.

Harris Benedict formula:

Women: BMR = 655 + (4.35 x weight in pounds) + (4.7 x height in inches) - (4.7 x age in years)

Men: BMR = 66 + (6.23 x weight in pounds) + (12.7 x height in inches) - (6.8 x age in year)

To calculate your daily calorie needs including exercise, multiply your BMR number from the above equation by the appropriate figure below:

If you are sedentary (little or no exercise): maintenance calories = BMR x 1.2

1. Light activity (light exercise/sports one to three days/week): maintenance calories = BMR x 1.375
2. Moderate activity (moderate exercise/sports three to five days/week): maintenance calories = BMR x 1.55
3. Heavily active (hard exercise/sports six to seven days a week): maintenance calories = BMR x 1.725

4. Extremely active (very hard exercise/sports and physical job or two times training): maintenance calories = BMR x 1.9

So for example, you are a thirty-four-year-old female who weighs 160 pounds, stands five feet four inches, and works out moderately four days per week. Your figures would look like this:

655 + (4.35 x 160) + (4.7 x 64)–(4.7 x 34) x 1.55 =
655 + 696 + 300.80–159.80 x 1.55
655 + 996.80–159.80 x 1.55
1651.80–159.80 x 1.55
1492.0 (BMR) x 1.55 (Activity quotient) = 2312.60 maintenance calorie intake

For weight loss, deduct 10 percent of your maintenance calorie intake from your maintenance calorie intake to get the appropriate caloric deficit:

2312.60 x .10 = 231.26 (caloric deficit)
2312.60–231.26 = 2081.34 (daily intake with deficit)

If you are not comfortable with the math calculations, there is a BMR calculator on our Web site (www.yourbodyyourlifey-ourself.com). You can now calculate with a certain degree of accuracy how many calories you should be consuming on a daily basis and can now divide this number of calories by the number of meals you will be consuming through the course of a day.

Understand that you will not have to do this at such an intricate level forever. However, it is very important that in the beginning stages of this process, you utilize this tool to gain an understanding of how quickly the calories can add up and what the portion size of your meals should be.

Making good quality choices in food/fuel is going to be as crucial as the quantity that is consumed. Consider a good nutritional choice would fit within some fairly basic parameters. Quantity and quality being the primary factors that dictate whether the food choice will be beneficial to your body's energy and nutrient needs or will bog down all of the life processes. Just a little further along, I will actually give you an extensive list of good nutritional choices and then arrange them in a sample meal format with meal timing to give you the best idea of what to eat when.

A good rule of thumb when making a decision of what you should eat is simply "fresh is best" and know that fresh cuts of lean protein, fresh fruits, and vegetables (organic is optimum), as well as freshly prepared beans and grains will provide your body with the highest quality fuel source. Your body is a lot like your car, and if you put poor-quality gasoline in your car, it runs poorly and could harm the engine; just the same principal applies to putting poor-quality food into your body.

We have all heard the term *moderation*, but what does that really mean? For some moderation might mean getting a monster order of fries in lieu of the *super* monster size, where with others moderation might be seen as cutting a normal meal portion down by a third.

The moderation principal is a good starting place in the lifestyle change process, helping to facilitate a sustainable habit (which is the whole point). One great way to begin this process is to take a normal portion of a given meal and cut it down by half then double the water intake for that meal. Also change the pace at which you eat (if you're a fast eater) to where you eat much slower and you focus on thoroughly chewing each and every bite and finish your water intake before you finish your food.

This will do a couple of things for you, one of the most important in this process as this is the first step in digestion and will allow your digestive system to better break down food components for nutrient distribution. The other is it will aid in overall satiety, as your stomach will have time to communicate to your brain that you are getting sufficient energy and trigger your "fullness" response much quicker.

The next step is to make it a goal to only consume foods whose ingredients you can pronounce. This is no joke; your body is designed to break down and utilize clean, unprocessed, and unaltered foods only. We were not designed to break down and metabolize/utilize shelf stabilizers, color enhancers, flavor enhancers, preservatives, additives, and any of the other hosts of chemicals that find their way into many common foods.

For instance consider that aspartame turns into formaldehyde in your digestive system. Absolutely nothing good can come from intentionally consuming poison (same principal applies to smoking and alcohol). This is just one small example of the toxic effects that food additives have on your body.

For all intents and purposes, you should begin your journey with a more conscious mindset of just what it is that you are consuming and the effects that it has on your body. Do not assume that just because it is being sold as food that it just has to be good for you—wrong!

Poor nutritional choices can be defined fairly easily as many of us are far too familiar with these already. The majority of instant, manufactured, and processed foods all fit into the category of poor nutritional choices. "But aren't they edible? Why do they sell them then?" Questionably yes, but do they supply our bodies with the clean, wholesome nutrition necessary for it to operate efficiently and maintain good health and body composition? Unfortunately most fall way short and have maximal profitability in primary focus, not your nutritional needs. So, with this, if it comes in a box, a bag, or premade from the frozen-dinners section, comes out of a drive-thru window, or has *instant* anywhere in the description, it is most likely not going to be a good nutritional choice.

Now think about this for a second. This little bit of information alone could be pivotal for you, and if applied, you could start dropping the pounds, increase energy levels, save money, and feel better over all with just this step alone! Look at making this change as a positive in your life, not as though you are taking something good away from yourself. Trust me; there is no deprivation in giving up junk food.

Another major pitfall in our modern world is the restaurant. From the fast-food mega chains, down to the small mom and pop country-cookin' spots, most all share the same focus as the processed-food manufacturers, profit, and marketability. I know that it may surprise you, but when a new dish is in the development phases at most restaurants, the chef is not sitting down with his nutrient data information sheets counting calories, fat, carbohydrates, protein, and a complete vitamin/mineral breakdown as the primary focus in his recipe development.

This chef is working on flavor profiling, texture components, and presentation (marketability). He is also working on creating this dish with maximal profit potential by using the best ingredients with the lowest cost. As much as I hate to admit it, your nutritional needs are not as high of a priority to them as your money.

A positive approach to eating out at restaurants is to make informed decisions about what is on the menu. A great starting place is to study the nutritional data for the restaurant prior to going. This will right away let you know what is a good choice and what may just sink you for the day. Some basic tips to follow when going out to eat are:

- If it swims in a vat of fat (deep frying), *I probably should not eat it.*
- If it is glazed, *I probably should not eat it.*
- If it is smothered in a cream or cheese sauce, *I should not eat it.*
- If it is topped with sour cream, cheese, or guacamole, *I should not eat it.*
- If I know that it is not lean, low fat, and is extremely high in calories, *I should not eat it.*
- If the word *butter* is mentioned in the description, *I should not eat it.*
- If the word *smothered* is anywhere in the description, *I should not eat it.*

There is no law that says you have to finish your meal in one sitting; take some with you to enjoy the next day. This is actually how you get the most for your money. Two meals—one price!

Vegetables, vegetables, vegetables, they are not only nutrient dense, they are quite filling.

I know many of you are thinking, *Well, good grief then, what do I eat?* The truth, whether you like it or not, is that you should eat just as responsibly at a restaurant as you would any other time.

You can enjoy the experience of dining out without totally gorging yourself on foods that are not only unhealthy but may make you feel pretty sick if you've been eating clean for a while.

The prime rule of the day is to simply be responsible and know that if you stick to your guns that you are more likely to not only feel better physically but you will also feel accomplished knowing that you have defeated yet another challenge that has crossed your path.

Having a "cheat" meal once every other week at a restaurant is not necessarily a bad thing and in many ways will give you something to look forward to, all the while stimulating your metabolism. You should just remember that an overindulgence can quickly go from reward to punishment, choose something you like but in a reasonable portion.

Another benefit of this practice is you will have the opportunity to learn to exercise discipline and become a little more conscious about the foods that got us on the "overweight" list to begin with.

Making food selections that fit the "healthy and nutritious" parameters that we are aiming for is going to present a fair amount of challenge and eye-opening experiences for you. With the "cheat meal," you will have a bit more flexibility to experiment with finding balance in indulgence and responsibility.

The following information is a very basic overview, with the purpose of pointing you in the right direction.

An area that may seem gray or abstract to some may be the choices in fats. Strange as it may seem, fat is a vital component to good health and must be included with a balanced diet. The key is to consume the right types of fats in the right quantities.

Believe it or not, by consuming the correct fats, not only will it *not* make you fat, you will actually store less fat! When your body senses that it is getting sufficient fat for its operational purposes, it will no longer look to store additional fat for essential function.

As a rule you will want to avoid the hydrogenated, partially hydrogenated, saturated, and trans fats. These guys are of the family of harmful fats that can not only be stored efficiently within your body (adipose and vascular plaque) but can also contribute to a number of other serious health risks.

The omega "family of fats" 3-6-9 as well as the monounsaturated and polyunsaturated fats are the types of fats that are beneficial not only to good health but also to weight loss. Some sources for these fats will be detailed in the foods list to follow.

I chose to place a bit of information about the fats here because there are so many confusing bits of sparsely researched data and fallacies that have made their way through the media and into the living rooms of the nation that there is a lot of confusion and misinformation about this crucial macronutrient.

The actual science goes much more in depth, being an entire book all to its own. However, for our purposes we want to give you enough solid information about a very crucial component to enable you to make an informed decision.

I have created a couple of lists of foods that I used during my weight loss and now during my maintenance that have given me excellent results and are nutritionally sound. Hopefully you will see the direction in which I am going with this and understand how your eating habits can be modified to get you on track.

Here are some awesome options that will help you in determining healthy and nutritious alternatives from the foods that have contributed to our health and weight problems.

Proteins:
- Chicken breast
- Fresh fish
- 93% or leaner beef
- Lean veal
- Turkey breast
- Lentils
- Lamb
- Soy products
- Tofu
- Egg whites
- Nuts (walnuts, peanuts, cashews, macadamias, almonds)
- Peanut butter in small portions (all natural is best)

Carbohydrates:
- Brown rice
- Pasta (whole wheat)
- Oats, Cream of Wheat, Kashi
- Breads (Whole grain, whole wheat)
- Barley, millet, buckwheat

- Unsweetened ready to eat whole grain cereals (natural granola is best)
- Sweet potatoes (baked with cinnamon, YUM!)

Fruits and vegetables:
- All green leafy vegetables (fresh only!)
- Colorful vegetables (fresh only!)
- Fresh fruits (melons make a great low cal snack!)
- Freshly squeezed (by you) fruit juice
- Plain frozen fruits and vegetables are occasionally ok
- Chilies and peppers

Fats:
- Extra virgin olive oil
- Walnut oil
- Fish oil
- Flax oil/meal
- Canola oil

Dairy:
- non-fat/low fat milk
- non-fat/low fat cottage cheese
- non-fat/low fat yogurt (sucralose/splenda sweetened is ok)
- Soy milk
- Rice milk
- Low fat ice cream occasionally
- Fat free sour cream
- Reduced fat 2% or less cheese

Miscellaneous:
- Salsa (fresh is best but jar is ok)
- Fat free salad dressing (beware of high sugar in some)
- Fat free popcorn

- Smart balance butter spread
- Sugar free jellies/jams (sweetened with Splenda)
- Splenda sweetener (made from sugar)
- Fat free mayonnaise
- Mrs. Dash is the "queen" of seasonings!

Beverages:
- Water (this is the most crucial and beneficial hydrating agent)
- Green tea
- Small amounts of coffee
- Avoid alcohol (this not only causes metabolic issues, but a long list of other inhibitive problems as well, also contains 7 empty calories per gram)

Here are some basic guidelines for deciding whether or not a food item fits the way that you want to eat for good health and weight loss.

Ask yourself these questions:

- Do my fruits and vegetables come in a can or box? *Fresh is best!*
- What else is there besides meat in this can? *Only fresh meats!*
- Are there any ingredients on this box/package I do not understand? *If there are, avoid them!*
- What is this exactly that I'm consuming? *If you do not know what it is, do not eat it!*
- What is the nutritional value in vending-machine food? *Most vending-machine food is junk; do not eat it!*
- It says "all natural," "reduced fat," "Omega-3," so it's got to be good, right? *Beware of the marketing,*

read the label, and if it contains anything that you do not recognize or understand what it is, do not eat it!

This is a very comprehensive list and should be a great starter to get you on the right path to making better nutritional choices. Understand that knowledge is power, and this power will make the difference in your success or failure in this process.

Each thing that you eat should be a conscious decision and you should understand that your purpose of eating is to supply your body with energy; nothing more, and nothing less.

Though it may be a challenge for some, preparing your own food is the most optimum scenario for making good nutritional choices. With a little practice and guidance, you will quickly discover that there are many ways in which you can make delicious meals that are nutritious and practical for your lifestyle.

One great technique that helps me out a lot is the "utility meat" concept. I will season and cook (grilling, roasting/baking, rotisserie, etc.) a large volume of meat (chicken, turkey, salmon, lean beef or lean pork, etc.) and then once cooled will cut and portion into small storage bags for later use. This concept works great for creating sandwiches, salads, stir-fry, main entrée, or any number of other combinations, quickly and cost effectively.

The utilization of plastic storage containers is highly valuable when preparing meals for the busy work week. You can use them for everything from snacks, lunches, and even entrée meals. This time sacrifice will be well rewarded not only in your waist line but also in your wallet!

What are the best ways of preparing these foods? For meats, the most potentially flavorful is grilling over a charcoal/wood fire. However, the methods of roasting, broiling, baking, and steaming are all fine as long as no additional fats are added or kept to a bare minimum. Season with any number of salt-free seasoning blends to taste.

Vegetables are tricky, as they contain many heat-sensitive nutrients, which means that maybe a very light steaming (still firm) or a light sauté would be okay. You never want to cook vegetables to "mush" or boil them, as this damages their nutrient value, and to be honest with you, kills their natural flavor. Veggies can be best flavored and seasoned with fresh herbs and spices, as this really brings out the natural flavors without adding additional sodium or calories.

There is an increasing number of cookbooks and Web sites (eatbetteramerica.com, for instance) that are now specializing in healthy recipes and helping to create lower calorie meal options without sacrificing flavor. Look for recipes that have complete nutritional data listed per serving with the recipe, and look for balanced (60 percent carbohydrate, 30 percent protein, 10 percent fat) meals. This percentage ratio applies to most meals as a "balancing" quotient; however specific macro-nutrient ratios can best be determined professionally based on your individual needs.

There is a lot of information in this chapter, and believe me this is only the tip of the nutritional iceberg. The human body is an enormously complex machine and the specific processes involved with intricate nutrition science are mind boggling! So, I have decided to only include what is most relevant and useful to accomplish your goals safely and efficiently without bogging down in the confusing science that many may find daunting and discouraging.

Some of the basic scientific information provided below is for your reference, giving you an idea of the basic values and metrics associated with the foods we eat.

A simplified definition of a calorie (kcal) is a unit of heat (through food in this instance) to heat one thousand grams water by one degree Celsius. Essentially, a calorie is a thermo-based energy unit that our bodies utilize for fueling our vital life processes. Because fats are most dense in calories, our body stores additional energy stores as lipids within adipose tissue and various other receptor points within our bodies.

What is important about this is the fact that your body sees calories as pure energy and will make every effort to retain what it cannot readily expend. This is why having a basic understanding of caloric content of food as relative to intake is very important to maintaining/reaching a healthy body composition.

Protein contains four calories per gram, carbohydrate contains four calories per gram, fat contains nine calories per gram (that is no typo, high-fat foods are *very* energy dense), and alcohol contains seven calories per gram (alcohol can create a host of metabolic challenges when you are trying to lose weight). Because alcohol use not only leads to liver disease and compromised cardiac function in addition to compromised metabolism, I strongly recommend this being among the habits you work to eradicate.

Macro nutrients are your proteins, carbohydrates, and fats. Micronutrients are your vitamins and minerals. The majority of your micronutrients come from your fruits and vegetables and are most densely provided in those with the darker colors.

To the contrary of many popular diets (one of which

the originator has died at an early age; RIP, good doctor), your body's first and most preferred source for fuel is actually carbohydrates. This means that carbohydrates (unless directed by a nutrition professional or your physician) should never be totally eliminated from your diet. Some food for thought: Fat is burned in a carbohydrate-fueled fire. No kidding!

The great secret to weight loss and reaching that ideal body composition is knowledge and balance. The commercial weight-loss industry would not want you to know this because you would no longer be in the market for their latest goofy gadget or pill. Knowing how to make a good decision and implementing this practice on a consistent and sustainable basis is the key to prolonged success for life!

I hope that you have found the information thus far in this chapter informative and helpful. I wish that I could say that losing weight, looking good, and feeling great also allowed for us to eat as much as we want of whatever we want. That is just simply not the case. In all actuality, if you want to lose the weight and get the results that will leave you looking and feeling the best of your life, you will have to make the nutritional adjustments.

Now that we have a bit of information about the components of a nutritious meal, just what defines a meal? The most simple definition would be, "A meal is a prepared quantity of balanced (generally: 60 percent carbohydrate, 30 percent protein, 10 percent fat) foods for the nutritional purpose of supplying energy for a given time." Okay, so what are we saying here? Each meal should consist of a protein, fat, carbohydrate (early in the day), vegetables, and fruit source in balanced proportions.

I am going to give you some examples of what meals should look like in the weight-loss process. Obviously there are going to be some components that are subject to change for each individual. However, this list will point you in the right direction as far as component selection, timing, and quantity are concerned.

The following information is merely suggestive, but it does fall perfectly in line with many of the foods that I ate during my weight-loss process and continue to eat for maintenance.

Some examples of what healthy meals would look like might be:

Breakfast meals:
Example 1:
1c whole rolled oats with 1/8 c craisins
2 boiled eggs
1c fat free milk

Example 2:
1 whole wheat English muffin w/fat free cream cheese
2c protein smoothie

Example 3:
1 ½ c scrambled egg beaters
2 pieces whole wheat toast
1 tbsp sugar-free jelly/jam
1c fat free milk

Example 4:
2 6-inch whole wheat pancakes
1/4c sugar free (Splenda sweetened) syrup
1 small slice low fat ham
1c orange juice

Example 5:
1 ½ c Whole grain cereal
1c fat free milk
¼ c almonds

Snack options:
Example 1:
1c fat-free cottage cheese
½ c fresh berries

Example 2:
1 medium sized apple
1 tbsp natural peanut butter

Example 3:
6 – 8 whole wheat crackers
2 slices reduced fat cheese

Example 4:
½ c fat-free/reduced fat yogurt
¼ c low fat granola

Example 5:
¼ c nuts (almonds, cashews, peanuts, macadamias)

1 medium piece fresh fruit

Lunch/dinner options:
Example 1:
6 oz baked/grilled salmon
1 ½ c steamed broccoli

Example 2:
5oz hamburger steak (93% or leaner beef)
¼ c mixed sautéd (trace oil) onions, green peppers, mushrooms
2 c green salad (mixed baby greens)
1 tbsp fat-free/reduced fat dressing (watch sugars)

Example 3:
4 oz meatloaf made with (93% or leaner ground beef)
1 ½ c mixed vegetables steamed

Example 4:
5 oz smoked pork loin
1 tbsp barbeque sauce
½ c steamed baby spinach

Example 5:
6 oz baked tilapia (seasoned with citrus seasoning)
1 ½ c steamed green beans w/pearl onions and herbs

If you noticed the trend in the composition of the meals, the majority of the carbohydrates are eaten early in the day (never eliminate carbohydrates from your diet unless advised by a physician or nutritionist). The general purpose of this is to prevent any radical increase in blood sugar/insulin levels during the most sedentary parts of the day.

In typical, most of us put out the majority of our work/activity load through the course of the day, thusly we need to fuel/refuel our body accordingly. However, as we prepare to wind down toward the latter portion of the day, our energy needs aren't as great, thus any starch/sugar consumption could induce the pancreatic response (increasing blood insulin levels) compromising our overall metabolic rate and facilitate efficient fat storage.

This technique works exceptionally well for those who have a day job. However, if you tend to work at night, the process works the same way just with a variance in your timing, by eating the high carbohydrate meals before work and the low/no-carbohydrate meals as you are approaching your time for rest.

Meal timing is also a crucial component in keeping the body running at peak efficiency/capacity. Many of you have heard the old "log on the fire" analogy as it relates to consuming food to fuel the metabolic fire. This is very true; however, I have a little different and more relatable analogy that will hopefully turn on the little light bulb above your head. "Hopefully you would not allow your car to run completely out of gas and stall on the side of the road before gassing it up would you?" This also applies to your body and the extremely complex engine that it is. If you wait until you get hungry to eat, that is the same as letting your car run out of gas before filling it up.

Studies show that people who eat only when they are hungry tend to eat many times more calories and have higher mean average body-weight/body-fat percentage ratios than those who eat small meals several times per day. You will also find that you will not feel deprived of food and in some ways feel as if you are eating more.

Ideal meal timing would include eating about every three hours or so, and a typical daily schedule might look like this:

6:00 AM	Breakfast
9:00 AM	Snack #1
12:00 PM	Lunch
3:00 PM	Snack #2
6:00 PM	Dinner/supper

> As a rule, regardless of what time you wake up, you want to consume a meal within an hour of waking and a small meal approximately every two and a half to three hours through the course of the day, up to three hours prior to going to bed.

This might look daunting if you currently only eat a couple of times per day or have a job that leaves time/resources at a premium. However, preparation, determination, and persistence are the keys to finding solutions to make this strategy work for you. Once you begin eating within this type of pattern, you will notice increased energy levels, diminished cravings and ravenous tendencies at meal times, and your ability to lose the weight will become much easier now that your body is no longer in a perceived state of famine.

Hydration is crucial not only for good health, but also in the process of losing weight. A simple rule for hydration is the "rule of eights." Consume eight ounces of water per hour during the day for eight hours (for an average adult). This process will not only help you to stay sufficiently hydrated, but will also aid in satiety.

Culinary planning and preparation can absolutely make or break the quality of a meal. One way to look at meal composition is like this. With the understanding that there are more than twice as many calories per gram (nine to be exact) for fat than there are for protein and carbohydrates (four each), then it stands to reason that you will be able to consume a larger portion of a given food that is lower in fat and stay within your calorie intake than you would a meal that is high in fat.

Oftentimes the foods we eat become fat laden in the preparation process, and the initial caloric density dramatically increased. There are a number of ways to get around this and still have food that is both appealing and nutritious.

Learning flavor profiling with various spices and herbs is a great way to add tremendous depth to the foods that you like (adding lemon pepper to steamed broccoli for instance) without having to smother that same piece of broccoli in butter or a fatty cheese sauce.

Grilling, roasting, baking, slow simmering, and rotisserie are all great ways of preparing protein sources (beef, chicken, fish, pork, etc.) and give you an excellent opportunity to introduce a lot of flavor into the party without bringing in tons of calories.

For instance, making a low-fat version of a chicken chili would simply involve combining the onions, peppers, beans, chicken breast chunks, spices, and low-fat/reduced-sodium chicken broth in a slow cooker or large pan on the stove.

Slow cook for a couple of hours, and you have an absolutely delicious and healthy meal choice for several servings.

Adding fresh fruit or using a small bit of fresh fruit juice to season salads is another fantastic idea to add flavor without introducing tons of empty fat and/or sugar calories (many from saturated sources).

Look for food components that are genuinely (watch out for creative marketing) reduced fat/low fat (i.e., reduced-fat cheese, fat-free sour cream, reduced-fat whole-grain crackers, etc.). By watching the fat intake of many of these meal components, you can save yourself a truckload of empty calories and will actually be able to consume a larger meal portion.

Please understand that I am not advocating elimination of fat from your diet entirely at all. As a matter of fact, using some fat like that from extra-virgin olive oil for sauté or stir-fry in small portion not only facilitates that cooking process, but is among the fats that are beneficial to you and essential for good health. Nuts such as almonds, cashews, macadamias, and walnuts are also very tasty meal components and also have great health benefits.

Read the labels and understand that not all fats are bad; however, you want to restrict the sources and quantities of these fats only to those that are essential, understanding that there are thousands of foods and meal components on the market that contain high fat calories from saturated, hydrogenated, and trans-fatty sources (regular milk, regular sour cream, regular cheese, regular ground beef, dark-meat chicken or turkey, potato chips, snack cakes, cheese sauces/spreads, regular salad, anything deep fried, dressings, lard, vegetable oil, regular mayonnaise, cream sauces, and the list goes *way* on!).

Understanding that food prepared with a little creativity and a consciousness in composition can not only taste great, be satisfying, but also be very healthy for you and aid in reaching those weight-loss goals. Eating healthy does not mean deprivation by any means; rather learning to eat healthy will allow you to explore a more mature enjoyment of what you eat.

For those of you who skip breakfast, this is an extremely bad idea on many fronts, hampering your weight loss and maintenance process significantly. It is just as it sounds "breaking the fast." As your body has rested through the night in slumber, it is now time to assemble its resources to get you through the day ahead. If these resources are insufficient, so will the available energy and capacity. With this, your ability to perform is compromised and so is your metabolic rate and ability to burn calories efficiently.

If this shoe fits, please try to make the effort to correct this habit. The rewards far outweigh the sacrifices of an additional few minutes in the morning. Preparation in this area will make adjustments much easier, so maybe pre-portioning out foods and storing them for quick on-the-go distribution may be in order to make it work for you.

Something that you must understand is that you are not only trying to lose weight; you are trying to lose fat. To accomplish this, the nutrition must be as close to ideal as possible (in concert with the exercise). Diligence and willingness to learn in this area will be well rewarded. There are a number of online and printed resources that will help you to understand much more of the science involved with nutrition. I strongly recommend that you take advantage of some of these resources. Knowledge is power, and power is success.

By learning some of the scientific principals behind human nutrition and the specific (founded on science) benefits of organic foods, herbs, antioxidants, phytonutrients, and how your body uses each component, you will learn how to make the best nutritional choices for your goals and lifestyle.

Hiring a good nutritionist/dietician at some juncture would be money well invested. These professionals will give you the customized planning and processes necessary to assure your results, as well as addressing any specific issues related to nutrition (diabetes, food allergies, chemical intolerances, etc.). They will also provide you with an empowering education that will help you to stay healthy for the rest of your life!

OH YEAH, IT'S EXERCISE TIME!

You did not think that I was going to write a book about weight loss and not include one of the most crucial components, did you? I know some of you may be breaking out in an allergic rash about now because you despise exercise. However, believe it or not, exercise is mostly a state of mind and actually has more to do with motivation and emotional drive than exertion and can stimulate the best of highs—the endorphin rush!

Venturing into an exercise program does not insinuate that you have to feel as if you are going to experience death by treadmill. Though the purpose of exercise is to evoke body-changing stimulus, take comfort in knowing that this does not mean that you must push to the brink of exhaustion every workout in order to reach your goals.

A well-designed and consistently-executed exercise program will not only guarantee you results on an enormous proportion physically, you will find that you mentally and emotionally will feel better through the process as well.

By design, the human body is one of the strongest and most amazing machines on the planet, with a capacity for work that is mind boggling! Understand that physical activity and labor is seen as just that by your body, not exercise. The human body is among the most adaptive organisms on the face of planet earth, and in order to make change, the body must constantly receive progressive stimulus.

You've seen it before in this book, and you're about to see it again. Get your physician involved before beginning any weight loss, nutritional, or exercise program. This is not optional and should be a first step.

It is also at this juncture that I must advocate that you get a professional fitness assessment by a certified professional. Exercise is an extremely complex process that involves enormous variables (seen and unseen) that can not only have direct effect on the weight-loss process but can have significant adverse impact if not done correctly.

Many fitness centers and personal trainers offer this service at little or no charge and can provide enormous insight into just what all is involved with getting you started in a structured exercise program safely and effectively.

Working with a personal trainer initially through this process is the absolute ideal scenario and could save you a lot of time and frustration. I know that this resource is not available to everyone (sure was not available to me at the time either) and that the financial commitment can be extreme. However, the education, compliance, and accountability components can be priceless!

If you are working with a health and fitness professional, you may skip ahead to other sections of this book that you find relevant; otherwise, please understand that even though I am a certified and degreed professional, each person is different and the information in this chapter is meant to be generalized and informative rather than a structured program.

Otherwise we will take you through a general assessment and let you gather the initial data that you need in order to begin designing an efficient and effective exercise program, safely.

Now, with that said, we need to understand that exercising regularly not only will help you to reach your weight-loss goals quicker but will also help to ensure that the weight you are losing is fat and not muscle.

Many women fear the all mighty m-word (muscle), as they feel that by strength training (lifting weights) that they might get "buff" or grow large, bulky muscles. This is far from accurate and must quickly be dismissed. You will learn further along that not only is strength training an essential component to your weight-loss success, it will help to give you a very pleasingly nice, lean/toned appearance. Through the course of this chapter, I will explain to you how strength training will not only not "bulk" you up (unless that is your goal, and you will need a different book for that), it will actually help you to reach your weight loss goals faster and more efficiently, with a much more desirable result at the end.

Another common misconception is that you can do "spot" training (i.e., crunches for a flat stomach) in order to address problem "fatty" areas. Unfortunately that is just simply not the case. The best way to lose the annoying belly fat and to get those shapelier thighs has nothing to do with the number of crunches you do or how many hours you spend riding the latest infomercial gadget. The best way to achieve these results is through full-body programming, combining both cardio respiratory and strength training.

A postural assessment should also be done and any postural misalignment/maladies be addressed through corrective exercise. This is something that a health and fitness professional can do for you, or you can have this done with recommendations by your primary physician.

Assessment is the starting place for any exercise program once given the medical go-ahead, and if you do not have the option of working with a fitness professional, we will take you through the basic steps of a standard fitness assessment. You will have to determine your starting place and have some base-line numbers to build upon for your programming.

It is important that you do not skip this step and just jump right into lifting and/or onto a treadmill. In order for you to exercise safely and with a sense of direction and balance, it is crucial that the baseline numbers be established first. Also, in the event that you have any strength imbalances or postural maladies (discovered through assessment), in order to prevent serious injury, you must consult with a professional or research how best to address these through the course of your programming.

At my studio we conduct a cardio-respiratory endurance/ efficiency assessment, upper-body strength (both push and pull), lower-body strength (squat) assessment, and a core (much more than just your abs) strength assessment. With these numbers we can determine what the most appropriate path is to take our client toward their road of health and fitness.

The same principals apply to you as well. This means getting a heart-rate monitor and establishing what your cardio-respiratory efficiency/conditioning levels are. You can usually find these monitors at most large retail stores in the sporting goods section or at a number of online sources.

Determining your heart rate is done by:

- Subtract your age from 220; this is your maximum heart rate
- Multiply this number times .70; this will be your sustaining/continual cardio exercise heart rate
- Multiply your maximum heart rate by .90; this will be your peak training (or burst) heart rate
- Also check your heart rate first thing in the morning before you get out of bed; this is your resting heart rate.

Another way of looking at how to do this is:

- 220–age = maximum heart rate
- maximum heart rate times .70 = sustaining/continual cardio exercise heart rate
- maximum heart rate times . 90 = peak training (or burst) heart rate

These numbers are important as they will help you to benchmark progress and understand just where your actual exertion levels are as compared to your perceived exertion levels.

If you have not exercised in a while, you will discover that your heart rate may increase rather rapidly through the course of the cardio-respiratory assessment. Please make written notes in your journal of this, as you will need to work to show weekly progress in cardio-respiratory efficiency by steadily increasing work capacity with moderated heart rate.

It is important that you know the difference between perceived exertion and actual exertion is how the exercise at a given intensity makes you feel relative to your heart rate. Now, there are a number of factors that will play into your perceived exertion rate, and we need to understand these factors going into this.

First is your mental and emotional state. If you just flat do not like exercise, you do not want to do it, you do not see the value in it, or you just want to get through it rather than getting the most out of it, you are going to be miserable the whole time. This is a problem that you need to look at first-hand and determine what is important to you and understand that nothing bad comes from doing something good for yourself. And yes, exercise is good!

Second is your nutrition and hydration. It is going to be vital that your eating habits and hydration habits are consistent and optimized to get the most from your exercise. The carbohydrates you consume are stored in your liver and muscles for energy, and you cannot allow yourself to ever eat totally "carb free." Because your body is over seventy-five percent water and this includes your muscles, it is vital that you stay very well hydrated. This will keep all of your body's systems (neurological, muscular, skeletal, digestive, respiratory, cardiovascular, thermo-regulatory, and many others) working correctly and optimize your exercise.

Third is exercise selection and duration. By varying the different cardio-respiratory exercises that you do in conjunction with the duration and frequency, you will build continual tolerance to higher exertion exercises for a longer period of time.

In my gym, I use what I call my "exert-o-meter" to measure perceived exertion with my clients. It works on a figurative scale of one to ten, with one being asleep and ten being oh my gosh! You will find that if you will make mental note of your "exert-o-meter" feeling with your actual heart rate; it will give you a fairly accurate gauge for your exercise tolerance.

For the cardio-respiratory efficiency assessment, you should (based on your conditioning level) look at doing a quick/speed walk on varying (with inclines) terrain, on a treadmill at the gym, or using just a step. Work at a pace at which you are comfortable but growing in speed progressive for the first two minutes (basic warm-up), then start pushing yourself until your perceived exertion is about an eight or nine (reference "exert-o-meter"), then stop and read your actual heart rate.

Make record in your journal of what you did, how long, how far (if applicable), your heart rate, and your perceived exertion (exert-o-meter) level. This information is critical, so please be sure that you do not skip this step.

Next is the upper-body strength assessment. In controlled conditions we use a basic push-up for this assessment, and this can be used by you as well (contingent that you have no medical or physical issues preventing you from doing this exercise).

Now understand that this exercise does not necessarily have to be done on the floor and can be modified to fit your abilities, by using anything from a bench to just pushing off of a wall. Illustrations of a basic push-up will be included for reference in the back of the chapter and can be referenced for a basic understanding of this exercise.

Do as many push-ups as you can with good form, whether they be modified or standard form and record in your journal how many and how you did them.

The pulling or rowing exercise should be done with weights or can be done on a rowing-type machine at a gym. This exercise will give you an idea of your flexor strength, as you will need to balance your pushing strength training with pulling strength training.

Your results should be recorded in your journal with what exercise you did, how many, and with how much weight. This information will be used to help you with maintaining synergy between pushing and pulling exercises and determine if you have any strength imbalances. Examples of rowing exercises will be provided to you in the back of the chapter.

Lower-body strength can be assessed by performing a basic compound movement used in everyday life called a squat. Please understand that there are many variations of the squat and that not all of them require you loading up a massive barbell on your back, squatting as low as you can, then exploding the back end out of your shorts trying to get it back up.

For our purposes we will just have you do a basic squatting movement, holding good form and getting a feel for what the optimum mechanics for this exercise are. It is critical that you understand how to squat properly before attempting this exercise, as many have an unsafe habit of trying to initiate the movement with their knees instead of their hips.

Visualize that you are going to sit into a chair (and for all intents and purposes place a chair behind you for practice).

Then, place your feet just on the outside of your hips, trying to keep the feet pointed straight ahead, with weight on your heels. Now shift your hips rearward and initiate your decent with a sitting motion, while working to keep your back in a straight/naturally arched position.

I know that this may sound a little daunting, but I will include some illustrations in the back of the chapter to help you understand this concept and to learn proper technique.

Once you are able to squat with good form, begin an assessment set by getting into position and doing as many squats in one minute as you can with perfect form. Record this result in your journal to be used later.

Core strength is next. This is a concept that unfortunately many have misunderstood and has become a sore (quite literally) source of disappointment for many who are trying to lose weight and get into better shape. The "core" is often thought of as just the abdominal muscles, and is trained with doing crunches or worse by riding on one of those goofy "ab magic" machine/contraptions found on infomercials.

Your core is a comprehensive complex of muscles associated with giving your torso rigidity and support and includes everything from hip flexors and spinal erectors to obliques and shoulder girdle stabilizers. This means that there is much more to training these muscles than just doing a few crunches and that weight-loss results around the waist are not achieved by simply "working" your abs.

The core assessment is done with an exercise called a plank, or prone-iso-ab. An illustration of this exercise is also included in the back of the chapter and does include a modification for those who cannot perform the exercise at full extension.

The purpose of assessing core strength is to simply find out what your ability to support your structural integrity with good form through the execution of a movement is. Safety is extremely important when exercising, and you must completely understand all of the mechanics behind each and every exercise before you do it. With this, it is imperative that you have a feeling for your strengths and weaknesses and address the weakness first in succession.

The plank is to be held in a position that is comfortable, and you must remain perfectly still (*never* allow your hips to drop below shoulder level when doing this exercise!) while executing the exercise. You will want to time how long you can maintain perfect form and write this time down in your journal for further programming.

Just the assessment alone can be quite a workout, and please understand that even though it may seem tough the first few times (for what it's worth, it's exercise; it's supposed to be challenging!), it does become not only more tolerable; exercise can quickly become very enjoyable.

Exercise is proven to not only improve weight-loss potential but also increase bone mineral density (helping prevent osteoporosis), increase metabolism, radically decrease the chances of diabetes and hypertension, as well as provides emotional, psychological, and even sexual benefits.

There is virtually nothing bad that comes from a consistent exercise routine that is both progressive and challenging. The benefits are a whole separate book's worth, while there are virtually no drawbacks.

Now that we have all of this information from our assessment, what do we do with it? As a health and fitness professional, I would take this information and develop a progressive program utilizing a number of exercises with varied intensity and duration to create a progressive program that will not only help to burn significant calories but also address any postural maladies/distortions that may be present.

For you, my suggestion would be to pick up a book on strength training. There are several out there, and some searches online will also provide reviews for those which are helpful and beneficial rather than those that are just good marketing (the bodybuilding books). These books will give you ideas, tips, suggestions, and very proficient illustrations to help you in determining which exercises best suit your needs and goals.

Now wait a second, why would I recommend a completely separate book? This is because knowledge is power, my friend, and power equals success! The more you know, the more likely you are to have the understanding of what it takes to meet and exceed all of your goals.

There is no single be-all, end-all book for all things exercise, fitness, weight loss, nutrition, and everything else health-related. It is good for you to tap various resources in order to empower yourself with the information necessary to travel in the right direction.

You will also need to develop a basic understanding of program design, with a total body emphasis. Full-body workouts not only burn the most calories but they also are the most efficient means of total body conditioning.

Program design needs to follow the following parameters:

- Proficient (know what exercises are training what muscles)

- Progressive (never do the same exercise with the same intensity twice, add additional weight/reps each time)
- Challenging (do not look for the easiest exercises because they are easy)
- Appropriate (do not exceed your proficiency or goal scope)
- Safe (I cannot emphasize how important safety is in exercising)
- Functional (mechanized training just does not cut it for good results; train for how you live!) Most exercise machines isolate particular muscles and are appropriate for body building or rehabilitative training only. You can hurt yourself permanently on these things!

Exercise selection is extremely important for maintaining a synergistic strength balance between pushing and pulling muscles, so it is important that you keep this in mind when putting together a workout program. Also, understand that the modality you choose will make a significant difference in your overall result.

For instance, a mechanized chest press is an isolation exercise designed to just focus on the pectoral muscles and those muscles alone. Where as a dumbbell chest press on a stability ball not only works on the pectoral muscles but quickly becomes a full-body workout and trains the body in a naturally functional process utilizing upper-body strength, core strength, and lower-body strength simultaneously.

What I am saying is to pick exercises that may have a prime mover (large muscle group) component (like the dumbbell chest press) and rather than using a bench or a uni-planar machine, choose to do it standing at a functional cable stack, on a stability ball, on a bosu, etc. These exercises incorporate more muscles, thusly making you stronger faster, training your body to work as a cohesive unit, and burning more calories.

An example of an exercise program that combines strength training with cardio for an overall expedited result might look like this:

Monday:					
Exercise:	sets:	reps:	weight:	rest:	notes:
Cardio 5-minute warm up					
Push-up	4	10		90 sec	alternating hand width
Alternating lunges	4	20	15 lb	90 sec	keep perfect form
Ball db chest press	4	15	25 lb	90 sec	feet close
Ball db tricep extn	4	15	12 lb	90 sec	alternate single leg
Standing db shoulder press	4	15	20 lb	90 sec	single leg standing
Elliptical cardio		45 min			intervals 75% - 90% max hr
stretch					

Tuesday:					
Exercise:	sets:	reps:	weight:	rest:	notes:
Cardio 5-minute warm up					
Lat pull down	4	15	75	90 sec	variating hand width
Standing db rows	4	15	25 lb	90 sec	feet close
Ball squats	4	20	20	90 sec	variating foot position
Ball back extention	4	15	n/a	90 sec	arms in iron-cross position
Standing db bicep curl	4	15	20	90 sec	alt single leg standing
Treadmill cardio		45 min			hill climb 8% grade 4 mph
stretch					
Wednesday:					
Exercise:	sets:	reps:	weight:	rest:	notes:
Cardio 5-minute warm up					
Lunges	6	20	10 lb db	1 min	alternating legs

Free-standing squats	4	15		1 min	Focus on eccentric
Plank	4	1 min		1 min	1 min perfectly straight
Swiss ball transfers	4	10		1 min	keep back flat
Elliptical cardio		45 min			intervals 75% - 95% max hr
stretch					
Thursday:					
Exercise:	sets:	reps:	weight	rest:	notes:
Cardio warm up 5 minutes					
Elliptical cardio		45 min			intervals 75% - 95% max hr
Stair stepper		15 min			80% max exertion
stretch					
Friday:					
Exercise:	sets:	reps:	weight	rest:	notes
Cardio warm up 5 minutes					

Push-up	4	10		90 sec	alternating hand width
Single-arm db row	4	15	35 lb db	90 sec	flat back, squared hips
Split squats	4	10 per leg	15 lb	90 sec	use bench support
Ball db chest press	4	15	25 lb	90 sec	feet close
High-cable row on ball	4	15	50 lb	90 sec	
Elliptical cardio		45 min			sustained 80% max hr
stretch					
Saturday:					
Exercise:	sets:	reps:	weight:	rest:	notes:
Cardio warm up 5 minutes					
Box step-up	4	50		1 min	25 each leg, high step
Jumping jacks	4	50		1 min	consistent pace
Crunch with med ball	4	25	8 lb	1 min	alternate single leg
Side plank	4	30 sec		1 min	switch sides before rest

Spin bike cardio		45 min			intervals 75% - 95% max hr
stretch					
Sunday:					
Active rest!					

This workout program is just to give you an idea what you will be able to work up to, but also lays out a pattern of exercises that are progressive and balanced. Your individualized program will vary depending on your fitness level and any physical limitations that you may have.

Make your workouts challenging and fun. By combining the two, you will quickly discover that exercising can become among the most enjoyable parts of your life. You should use the numbers gathered in your assessment and work to build on those each week. Keep accurate records and reassess yourself every thirty days with the same assessment to record and note progress.

There is so much more that can be said about exercise and the intricacies of biomechanics, kinesiology, human-movement science, progressive programming, exercise physiology, and on and on. However, that is not what this book is about. This book is meant to get you pointed in the right direction and to give you the basic information necessary to start making changes for yourself.

On average a workout should not take any longer than about one hour from warm up to final flexibility. Keep the mindset that workout time is about business only, limiting the social interaction to post-workout times. You need to monitor your rest breaks between sets and exercises and know that prolonged rest is time wasted! In order to get maximal conditioning benefits and calorie expenditure, you will need to keep moving consistently with minimal rest.

Other means of exercise that can be worked into your programming can be things like yoga, Pilates, zumba, aerobics, etc. These things all have their place, but none are a completely comprehensive modality and must be used in addition to but not in place of strength training and cardio-respiratory training.

Do not forget stretching at the end of each and every exercise session. It is important to remain flexible to not only enhance your performance but also to prevent injuries. Static stretches work fine when doing this type of training. You want to select stretches that will allow you to completely stretch your full body after each workout.

When stretching, the following rules must be followed. Pull the muscles tight in a "regular" range of motion, avoid pulling at odd angles, and remember that pain is not the goal here. The muscles should be pulled tight but not painful. Hold each stretch about thirty seconds and repeat. Do not bounce when stretching. There is a "type" of stretching called ballistic stretching that can cause injury to your muscle fibers rather than providing a flexibility benefit, so to prevent the risk of injury avoid this method.

Do not get so caught up in the exercise process that you forget the value in rest. It is equally as important that you allow your body to recover from intense exercise by getting at minimum of eight hours quality sleep per night and not allowing yourself to train to pure exhaustion every workout.

Though intensity is important, it is equally crucial that you understand that more is not always better and that one of the most vital components in determining whether or not what you are doing is beneficial is to simply listen to your body.

Muscle cramps (different from stimulated soreness), fatigue, loss of appetite, lethargy, and lack of motivation can all be signs of overtraining. In the event you encounter this condition, you need to roll things back a bit. Take a couple of days off from the gym, go for a walk in the park or a casual bike ride instead, and let your body recover.

Done right, incorporating consistent exercise into your lifestyle will quickly become one of the most emotionally and physically beneficial things that you can do for yourself!

SAMPLE EXERCISES USING MINIMAL EQUIPMENT

Squat with Stability Ball

Legs

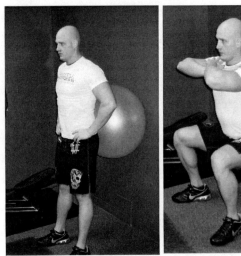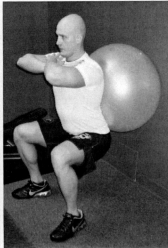

Place ball in the small of your back against a solid wall. Stand with feet slightly wider than hip-width apart and weight on your heels. Descend slowly in a "sitting" fashion until your hips are just shy of parallel with your knees. Slowly reverse direction, ascend, and begin again. This exercise can also be done with dumbbells and medicine balls for weight.

Lunge

Complete Legs, Core

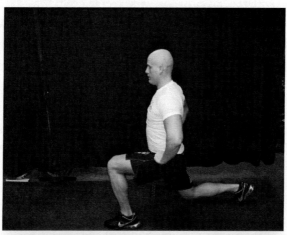

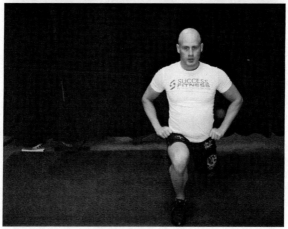

With your shoulders at neutral, chin level, feet hip width, core engaged, hands on hips, and back straight, begin by taking a long step forward. Once your balance is secured, initiate your descent by bending the back knee first and descend to an angle that is challenging yet comfortable. (Ninety degrees on each side is optimal.) Reverse direction by driving rearward with the forward foot while keeping your back straight. This exercise can also be done with dumbbells and medicine balls for additional challenge. One step per leg out and back to neutral is one rep.

Stability Ball Hamstring Curl

Core, Hamstrings, Hips

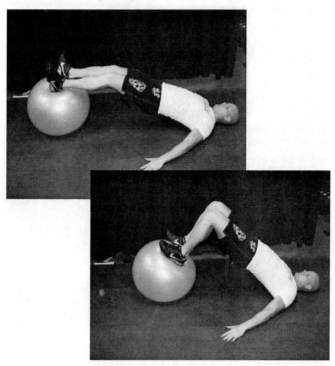

With your back flat, place your heels on the top of a stability ball hip-width apart, hands to the sides, glutes engaged (maintain through the entirety of the movement), and legs extended. Start position is a straight line from ankles to shoulders. To initiate the movement, bend the legs to a ninety-degree angle, allowing the ball to roll beneath your feet. Your feet should be flat on the top of the ball with your knees forming a straight line to your shoulders at the top of the movement. All the way in and all the way out is one rep.

Leg Extension

Core, Thighs, Shoulders, Hips

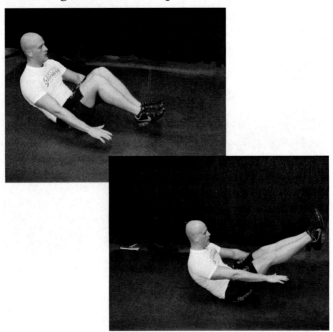

From a standard V-sit position, extend the legs to a completely straightened position to engage the quadriceps muscles (thigh muscles) while keeping the knees parallel with the center of your chest and back straight. Slowly bend the legs and reset for another rep. A medicine ball, dumbbell, or ankle weights can be used for added challenge.

Free Standing Squat with Dumbbells

Legs, Core, Biceps, Shoulders

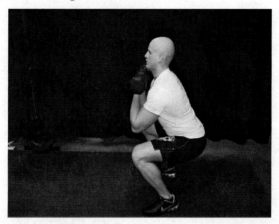

Choosing dumbbells of a manageable weight yet challenging, in a full-standing position, bring the dumbbells to a front-load position with palms facing and close to your body, keeping shoulders in a neutral position. Space feet just wider than shoulder width, back straight, and engage your core. Shift your weight to your heels and slowly descend in a sitting motion, shifting the hips first. Focus on keeping strict joint alignment, never allowing the knees to travel inward or outward from the ankles. Hips should not drop below parallel with the knees. Ascend in the same manner, keeping your weight on your heels, and repeat to complete one rep.

Medicine Ball Overhead Squat

Legs, Core, Shoulders

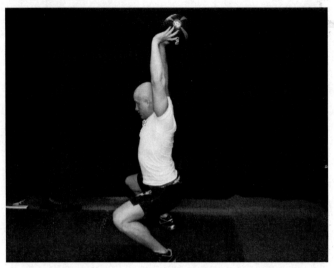

Choose a medicine ball of manageable but challenging weight (a dumbbell will suffice as well), with your arms fully extended and load directly above your shoulders. Space feet just wider than shoulder width, back straight, and engage your core. Shift your weight to your heels and slowly descend in a sitting motion shifting the hips first. Focus on keeping strict joint alignment, never allowing the knees to travel inward or outward from the ankles. Hips should not drop below parallel with the knees. Ascend in the same manner, keeping your weight on your heels, and repeat to complete one rep.

Stability Ball Transfer

Core, Hips

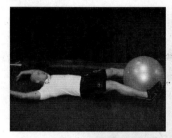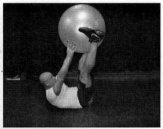

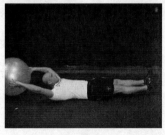

Begin lying flat on your back with legs extended, Swiss/stability ball between your ankles. With your arms extended over your head, slowly elevate both your feet and hands simultaneously by contracting your abdominals. Elevate both the hands and feet until you are able to reach the ball; at this point slowly reverse direction bringing the ball directly behind your head and feet straight out without touching the ground, reverse direction to complete one rep.

Bench Push-up

Chest, Core, Shoulders, and Triceps

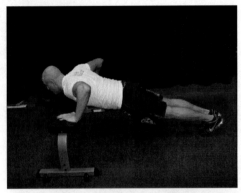

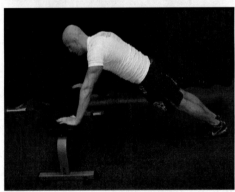

Utilizing a bench or a pair of chairs, place your hands just wider than shoulder width, keeping your back straight, begin your descent from a fully extended position. Slowly bend the arms until a ninety-degree angle is reached and reverse direction. This is one rep.

Standard Push-up

Chest, Core, Shoulders, and Triceps

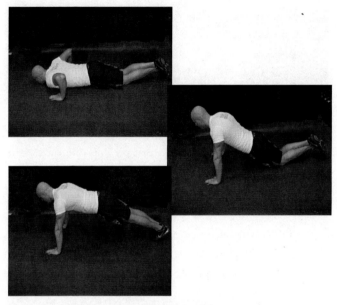

Begin at a fully extended position either on your toes or on your knees (based on your strength abilities) with your arms just wider than shoulder width. Descend slowly until your arms reach a ninety-degree angle, then reverse direction completing one rep.

Free Standing Dumbbell Row

Middle-upper Back and Biceps

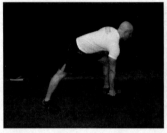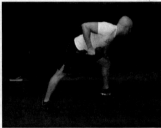

Begin with a split stance (foot forward opposite of the arm you are rowing with), hips square and back straight. Place the elbow of the non-pulling arm on the thigh of the forward leg for support. With a dumbbell of moderate weight in the pulling hand, execute a motion similar to reaching for the floor, then raising the elbow toward the ceiling. All the way down and back up is one rep. Reverse the process to switch sides.

Romanian Dumbbell Dead Lift

Lower back, Glutes, Hamstrings, Core

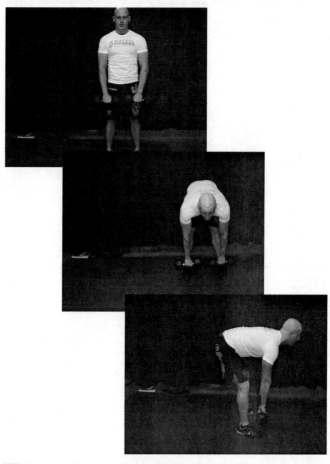

With a moderate weight dumbbell in each hand, begin standing up straight with good posture, feet just wider than shoulder-width apart. With just a slight bend at the knees, slowly begin your descent at the hips, while keeping your back in a straight (naturally arched) position. Allowing the weights to hang beneath the shoulder, descend to just shy of parallel to the ground. Ascend slowly, engaging your glutes and keeping your strict posture, pulling the shoulders to neutral at the top. This completes one rep.

Stability Ball Back Extension with Iron Cross

Glutes, Low Back, Middle Back, Upper Back, Core

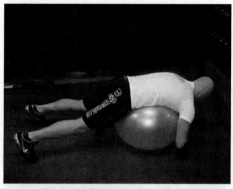

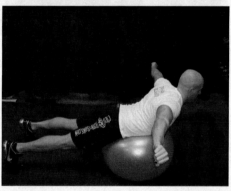

Lay on your stomach across the top of a stability ball, finding your center balance point. Space your feet just to the outside of your hips and allow your body to roll over the top of the ball. Slowly ascend, pulling your back into a slightly arched position, keeping your neck straight, and bringing your arms out to the sides with wrists parallel to the shoulders. Squeeze your shoulder blades together and hold for five seconds then slowly descend. This completes one rep.

V-sit

Core, Lower Back, Hips, Shoulders, Legs

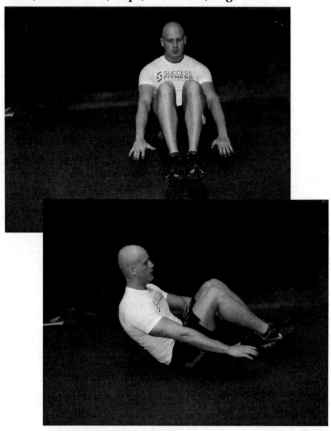

Seated with back straight, knees bent toward chest with feet elevated, bring your chin level and arms out to the side of your body close to the legs and hold this position with good form for timed repetitions.

Russian Twist

Core, Hips, Legs, Lower Back

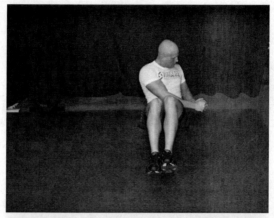

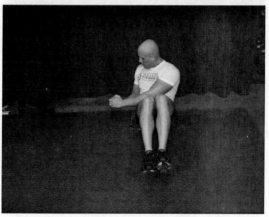

From a standard V-sit position (seated with back straight, knees bent toward chest with feet elevated), clasp your hands together, and with a smooth rotation of the shoulders, rotate your torso and lower your hands toward the floor, alternating left to right. One rotation to each side equals one rep.

Plank

Total Body Core Builder

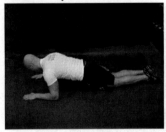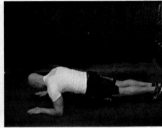

Based on your strength and body type, this exercise can be done in standard form or in modified form. Begin lying on the floor, placing your elbows directly beneath your shoulders and elevate your body off of the ground in a perfectly straight (good postural alignment) line. Standard form will have you straight on your toes while modified will have you on your knees. Hold for a determined period of time for one set. Do not allow your hips to drop below your shoulders. You must stay as still as possible to get maximum benefit from this exercise. You may also change up this exercise by straightening your arms to a fully extended position and holding, to recruit more of an upper body component.

Superman with Iron Cross

Upper Back, Lower Back, Glutes, Hamstrings, Neck

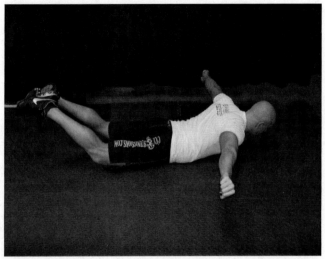

Lying on the floor on your stomach, slowly elevate your upper and lower body simultaneously while keeping your abdomen flat on the floor. Raise your arms out to the sides with wrists parallel to the shoulders and squeeze your shoulder blades together. Hold this position without movement for a determined period of time to complete one set.

Get creative with exercise and do not be afraid to try new things. By using bands, balls, free weights, free-motion cables, and body weight as your exercise modality, in lieu of machines, your workouts will be much more productive, safer, more challenging, and more fun!

ACCOUNTABILITY: YEP, YOU HAVE A SNITCH

One of the biggest components of what I do professionally has to do with accountability. I hold my clients responsible for being to their sessions on time and as scheduled. Additionally we have a system put into place to monitor body composition and weight. This allows for us to corroborate our client's journals with their actual numbers to assure us that the information being recorded is both accurate and in compliance with trainer instructions.

When beginning this lifestyle change process, you will be no different, as you will need to have systems in place that are beyond your direct control to help you stay accountable.

With this, you will need to contact a close friend, coworker, or relative and share with them what it is that you are doing and what you want to accomplish. This will not only help to keep you on track with your record keeping and overall results but will also give you an avenue of support for those times when it's not so easy to stay on track.

This person should be present to weigh you once per week, recording the numbers in your journal themselves, and to review your journal. It is so easy to fudge a little here and there when you are policing yourself, but it can quickly become a different creature when someone else is playing the "big brother" role.

I know that it's easy to come up with a thousand and one reasons (or excuses) why this may not work for you; however, you must understand that this person is not there to criticize you or to judge you. They are there for the sole purpose of supporting you and giving you the encouragement that it takes to move forward.

I had a tough time with this one and wound up policing myself. However, because I had so many friends, family, and coworkers watching my progress, I knew that I had to remain really diligent in order to keep from disappointing so many people. This gave me the strength and determination to stay regimented and to not allow myself to drift backwards.

If you have never kept a diary, this is a good time to start. A diary will give you an opportunity to vent and release any pent-up emotions that you may be dealing with, without resorting to food for comfort. Keeping a diary will also give you a written, chronological record of your progress and how you feel each day. Stuff that you may want to put in an entry may be: date, time, and mood. Then make mention of the challenges that you have faced for the day and then finish your entry with at least five good things that you have accomplished for the day. It is important to remain upbeat and positive through this process, especially in the onset.

Once you have adapted to the changes and everything

is becoming routine, you will see that the list of challenges associated with nutrition and exercise are diminishing, and the list of positive/good things for the day will increase. It's just really very exciting to see firsthand that your hard work has paid off through the course of time, and you have a permanent written record to reflect on how you arrived.

Compliance and accountability can become extremely difficult when faced with a lot of temptations on a regular basis. With this, it is important to limit your exposure to these temptations. This can be done by not buying unhealthy foods at the store and having them around you. Even though others in your family may enjoy these foods, you and they must understand that these things are no better for them than they are for you, and making healthier choices will pay off for all of you.

Another common place for many to falter is in the restaurants. I touched on restaurants a bit in the nutrition chapter but cannot reiterate enough how important it is to make these visits few and far between to reduce temptation.

I used to (and occasionally still do) have a "cheat" meal for lunch on every other Sunday as a reward for a great week. This will do a couple of things for you, the first being the satisfaction of feeling like you are not being totally deprived of all the things that you like. The other is the metabolic enhancement effect of consuming a higher-calorie meal than normal. It's true; your body will be thrown a curve ball by an occasional high calorie meal and will send your metabolism into hyper drive.

Now you need to understand that this is not a justification to throw down on a big meal every other day with the intention of "super charging" your metabolism. Unfortunately it does not work like that; however, this every other week indulgence will not only keep your emotions happy and spirits high; it will also help keep you dropping those pounds.

The reality is, no matter who you bring into this process and what other fail-safes you put into place, these things are only supplemental to the drive, motivation, and determination that can only come from your heart. Sure, making a significant lifestyle change is not going to be a walk in the park, but is it worth doing? Yes. Is it worth doing right? Of course!

This is a process that dictates that you will get out of it what you put into it. Work hard, stay smart, remain diligent, and accountability/compliance will be a "piece of cake!"

LONGEVITY: HOW TO MAKE IT STICK

There is so much that you have learned through the course of this book, from motivation, nutrition, and exercise through accountability. We now have to create a means in which to make all of this new stuff work for you, not just for now but forever.

Just how do you go about making such a significant shift permanent? Absolutely the very best way to make this happen is to get involved in a sport or activity that you thoroughly enjoy and stick with it in some capacity, begin early on and work up to full involvement. Even if your choice is something recreational like biking or hiking through nature trails, these things get you outdoors and keep you active. You will find that once engaged, the stresses of daily life seem to become less significant, and your quality of life becomes much better.

First things first, what is it that you like to do? Is it biking, gardening, tennis, swimming, or even football? There are any number of a thousand activities that may not require maximum exertion but keep you not only moving and active but really enjoying life. I strongly encourage you to actively seek out these activities and look to try new things and conquer new experiences. Though something as extreme as skydiving may be extreme for some, it can be a positive life-changing event for others.

A great example of how I have made significant change in my life lies in the fact that not only am I now a personal trainer, working long hours through the course of a day, but also an avid mixed martial artist, practicing Muay Thai, Brazilian Jujitsu, and Marine Corps martial arts. These things are not only great for self-defense, but make for an awesome workout too. In order to perform well in mixed martial arts, I also need to be regimented in both my strength training and my endurance cardio. This has allowed for me to be in the very best shape of my life!

There are days when I will get out of bed, look at myself in the mirror, and just be awestruck at what is looking back at me. It just amazes me at the difference in self-perception and the rejuvenated spirit that I get daily from having changed my life and permanently sustaining these changes.

Consider that at my heaviest, I wore a size four X T-shirt and a size fifty waist pants. I now wear a medium shirt (which shows off a muscular upper body and slim waist nicely), and a size thirty-four to thirty-six waist pants. It is just absolutely amazing to feel good about the way that I look to not only myself but also to others.

Where I'm going with this is you will quickly discover that once you are at your "maintenance" weight and body composition, you will never want to go back no matter what it takes. One of the best ways to keep from making the moves that begin the snowball plummeting down the mountain is the key elements that got you to the point where you discovered that you needed to make changes from the very beginning.

For many of us, the cause typically reverts back to emotional trauma or some sort of event in our lives that led us to turn to food for comfort. Once you have become fully accustomed to your change in lifestyle, you will discover that even when times are tough there are other ways to deal with the same issues that would have caused you to find comfort in food.

A good deal of sustainability will come from your attitude and approach to maintaining your motivation to keep diligent with healthy eating habits and exercise. If you reach a point at which you start to feel as if you are depriving yourself of something that you enjoy, take a look at the key elements of what it is about that item (nachos, cake, cookies, whatever) that evokes an emotional response of satisfaction. Then think about a non-food-related item that gives you that same sense of emotional fulfillment (playing a game, writing a poem, creating a painting, getting a massage, etc.) and then choose an alternate source for this fulfillment.

The truth is emotions do not burn calories, and our purpose for eating and making nutritional choices is not to satisfy our surface cravings. Rather, when you get into the habit of making smart choices in food and portion control, you will discover that binge eating is no longer a viable option for dealing with stress and anxiety, and you will feel accomplished for having found an alternate avenue to deal with daily issues.

Peer eating is another road on which you can quickly find yourself headed for a ditch. What I mean is finding yourself in a situation where you go out to eat with the family, on business, or just a social gatherings where food is the main attraction, and you're in the awkward position of trying to decide whether to potentially offend someone or stand out in the crowd by eating a small, limited amount of food, or do you just try to fit in by indulging?

This situation still falls under the same heading as everything else in this book, and that is balance. For instance, choosing to have some of the roast turkey, steamed carrots, and cantaloupe in lieu of the prime rib, garlic mashed potatoes, and baked Alaska for dessert. In making a conscious decision about what to eat and in what portions, you can quickly maintain your emphasis of keeping the event social, enjoying the company of others, rather than making the event about food and how to not stand out while avoiding going overboard.

There is absolutely nothing in this world worth surrendering all of your hard work and dedication for and allowing you to lose hard-fought ground. Every day of life is about moving forward, maintaining the understanding that you no longer have control over things that have happened in the past. However, there are many things in your life in the present and future you can influence through good attitude and positive thinking.

UM, WHAT THE?

In describing to you everything that I did in order to lose 177 pounds in just fifteen months, I mentioned that I did some non-conventional metabolic manipulation in order to continue making progress without plateau. This technique is vital because the human body is among the most adaptive organisms on planet earth and will quickly adapt to any continual stimulus (nutritional, environmental, exercise, or other) placed upon it.

In order to be successful with this technique, you will have to have been in complete compliance with the lifestyle change process for at minimum one month and have developed a complete understanding of how to calculate calories and macronutrient ratio percentages.

Once you have established this foundation, you will begin the metabolic manipulation process to avoid hitting any plateaus in your progress. How we keep things moving is by cycling, or periodization as it is otherwise known, in both nutritional intake and exercise. This will help to facilitate optimal weight loss and conditioning benefits; however,

I cannot stress enough that when employing this technique, you must follow it strictly and understand exactly what you are doing and why you are doing it.

The first component will be nutritional cycling. How this is done is by manipulating the macronutrient (protein, carbohydrate, and fat) intake as well as the caloric intake of your meals through the course of a week.

You will need to have your current intake numbers at hand as you go into the calculations, as these are needed to accurately calculate your daily intake.

Here's how it works:

Day 1:
Heavy exercise day (strength and cardio sixty minutes); keep calories and macronutrients at normal daily intake.

Day 2:
Moderate cardio day (forty-five minutes or less, seventy percent max intensity); subtract ten percent from your daily calorie intake, decrease carbohydrate intake by ten percent and increase protein intake by ten percent

Day 3:
Heavy exercise day (strength and cardio); increase total calories by ten percent from normal daily intake and increase carbohydrate intake by ten percent keeping other percentages normal (extra calories will come from carbohydrate sources)

Day 4:
High cardio day (sixty-minute interval) decrease overall calories by fifteen percent and increase carbohydrate by five percent

Day 5:
Strength training: increase calories by ten percent, increase carbohydrate by five percent, and increase protein by five percent

Day 6:
Active rest day: cycle calories back to normal intake, decrease carbohydrate by five percent increase protein by five percent

Day 7:
Active rest day: decrease calories by ten percent, decrease carbohydrate by ten percent

I know that at first glance this looks rather daunting and somewhat confusing. This is the point! Just as you are scratching your head, so will your metabolism, as it will not know what is coming next. We can simplify the process for you so that you can understand what to do; however, you want to continually leave your body guessing what is coming next.

Notice that on the higher exertion days the calories and the carbohydrate levels are higher. This is to facilitate glucose transport into your muscles to be used as glycogen for energy and support growth of lean-muscle mass, all the while stimulating your metabolism.

Because your body's need for "ready" energy is diminished on lower exertion days, the carbohydrate levels are brought down as well as the caloric intake. This will allow you to offset your calorie consumption with exercise displacement, forcing your body to burn more fat for energy on these days.

I know you may be thinking, well why don't we just stick to doing the whole thing this way because it will help burn more fat. The answer is because your body's nutritional needs will fluctuate with the demand placed upon it, and it will become necessary to accommodate these demands appropriately or your weight loss will come to a screeching halt!

As a general rule for most adults, also consuming sixteen ounces of pure water per hour for eight hours will help to keep your hydro-regulatory systems working properly and believe it or not will facilitate pure fat loss.

Water aids in lipid transport from adipose tissue, and when not provided to the body in sufficient quantities, water can also be retained by fat cells giving that "bloated/puffy" look to subcutaneous fat. Thusly further solidifying the necessity to remain well hydrated to fully utilize these techniques.

Understand that as your weight drops so does the amount of energy that you need to sustain your current body composition. As a basic rule, for every ten pounds that you lose, you will also want to cut your caloric intake by approximately ten percent in order to continue losing weight. Now this gets tricky the leaner you get and the more strength training that you do. It is important to never let your calorie intake ever go below around 1200 kcal. Your body must have sufficient calories in order for all of the systems to run appropriately and to sustain a healthy rate of energy metabolism.

This metabolic manipulation technique can be employed throughout the entirety of this process; however, you must remain diligent about keeping track of your calorie intake to make optimal progress.

Once you have reached the maintenance phase of your lifestyle change process, it will no longer be necessary to cycle your calorie intake, and you can calculate your maintenance calorie consumption by utilizing your current BMR. The Harris Benedict Formula is the most beneficial for this calculation, and it looks like this:

Women: BMR = 655 + (4.35 x weight in pounds) + (4.7 x height in inches) - (4.7 x age in years)
Men: BMR = 66 + (6.23 x weight in pounds) + (12.7 x height in inches) - (6.8 x age in year)

To calculate your daily calorie needs including exercise, multiply your BMR number from the above equation by the appropriate figure below:

If you are sedentary (little or no exercise): maintenance calories = BMR x 1.2

1.   Light activity (light exercise/sports one to three days/week): maintenance calories = BMR x 1.375
2.   Moderate activity (moderate exercise/sports three to five days/week): maintenance calories = BMR x 1.55
3.   Heavily active (hard exercise/sports six to seven days a week): maintenance calories = BMR x 1.725
4.   Extremely active (very hard exercise/sports & physical job or two times training): maintenance calories = BMR x 1.9

So for example, you are a thirty-four-year-old female who

weighs 160 pounds, stands five feet four inches, and works out moderately four days per week. Your figures would look like this:

$$655 + (4.35 \times 160) + (4.7 \times 64) - (4.7 \times 34) \times 1.55 =$$

$$655 + 696 + 300.80 - 159.80 \times 1.55$$

$$655 + 996.80 - 159.80 \times 1.55$$

$$1651.80 - 159.80 \times 1.55$$

1492.0 (BMR) x 1.55 (Activity quotient) = 2312.60 maintenance calorie intake

If you are not comfortable with the math calculations, there is a BMR calculator on our Web site. This will help to give you the most accurate numbers next to a clinical body composition analysis.

It is important to know that you do not have to stick to the "numbers" as a lifetime commitment. The idea is to give you a solid sense of what a balanced and reasonable daily intake should be, what food sources to choose, and when to eat. As creatures of habit, we thrive on consistency and systems. So even though the learning curve may be a bit laborious, the long-term process is actually quite easy.

PUTTING IT ALL TOGETHER

Who would have thought that a more realistic look at health, fitness, and weight loss would include so much information and variables? This short chapter will help you to summarize, analyze, and make sense of what you have just read then mix it all together into a practical way of life for you!

In the first couple of chapters, we addressed some of the basic "why should I do this" components, then we looked at the practical "how do I do this" in addressing nutrition and exercise. Finally we learned just how to make the entirety of this process permanent and sustainable.

Now let's look at practical application. For instance, you are a working housewife with three children (not including your husband) to look after, a long day of errands to run, and tasks to get accomplished, all on a tight schedule. How are you going to make all of this stuff work for you? Because it is not at all uncommon for me to work a twelve- to fourteen-hour day with little to no breaks, I can empathize with you and will share just exactly how I make it work.

Being a certified chef as well as a personal trainer, I have the privilege of making all of the meals for my family. I have found that one of the most efficient means of getting everyone fed a quality meal in the appropriate quantity and timing requires a little bit of planning but is not as difficult as it may seem.

Pick a day (weekends typically work best) to allocate at least two hours to food preparation. At this time you can pre-prepare a good deal of your proteins for the week (grilling fish, roasting chicken, smoking turkey breast, etc.). You then simply portion out each protein according to how it's going to be used (larger portions for family meals, smaller for individual meals). Most cooked meats will keep well in the refrigerator for four to five days safely. Any additional meats can be frozen and kept for several weeks.

Just this step alone saves a ton of time through the course of the week. Now, look at pre-portioning out other items in small airtight containers (cereal, yogurt, salad, fresh veggies, nuts, etc.). This will help to streamline your meal preparation and ensure that you (and everyone else) get your meals in time and quality.

A touch of irony is that this process/technique is actually more efficient, more cost effective, and easier to do than most current meal practices in the average American household. It just requires a couple of hours per week to make everything happen.

Set realistic goals for both weight loss and in exercise progression. Having or setting unrealistic goals/expectations is a seed for disappointment and can quickly squash all motivation to continue. An average weight loss would be between a pound and a half to two pounds per week, and a typical strength gain would be approximately five percent (per compound exercise) every two weeks.

Expect to have sore muscles, expect to sweat, expect to get a little tired, expect to make smarter nutritional decisions, expect results!

It does not require a degree in nutritional science, exercise physiology, or health sciences to live a healthy life and stay physically fit. The information provided within this book gives you a solid foundation of how your body works and what it takes to maintain it in optimum health. By simply utilizing this basic information in conjunction with some discipline and determination, you can achieve and maintain your lifestyle change for now and forever! I know this because I live it, I teach it, and it has become my passion to educate the world, re-gifting the gift of life!

GLOSSARY

Accountability–the acknowledgment and assumption of responsibility for actions. Encompasses the obligation to report, explain, and be answerable for resulting consequences.

Activity–something done as an action or a movement

Adipose tissue–connective tissue which stores fat and which cushions and insulates the body

Antioxidants–a group of vitamins that acts against the effects of free radicals

Aspartame–an artificial non-saccharine sweetener

Bariatric surgery–various surgical procedures performed to treat obesity by modification of the gastrointestinal tract to reduce nutrient intake and/or absorption

Bio-available–measurement of the extent of a therapeutically active drug that reaches the systemic circulation and is available at the site of action

Biomechanics–deals with the mechanics of the human or animal body, especially concerned with muscles and the skeleton

Body composition–describes the percentages of fat, bone, and muscle in human bodies

Bone mineral density–used to measure bone density and determine fracture risk for osteoporosis. It may also be used to determine how effective an osteoporosis treatment is.

Bosu–an athletic training device consisting of an inflated rubber hemisphere attached to a rigid platform. It is also referred to as the "blue half ball" because it looks like a stability ball cut in half. The name is an acronym which stands for "Both Sides Up."

Calorie–the amount of heat needed to raise the temperature of one gram of water by one degree Celsius

Carbohydrate–a sugar, starch, or cellulose that is a food source of energy

Cardio respiratory training–oxygen and carbohydrate fueled exercise (i.e., running, calisthenics, elliptical trainer, etc.) at sub-maximal capacity with the purpose of conditioning the heart and lungs as well as increasing the efficiency in which the body utilizes oxygen for fuel

Circuit training–a type of training in which strength exercises are combined with endurance/aerobic exercises, combining the benefits of both a cardiovascular and strength-training workout

Cleansing supplement–a nutritional supplement utilized for the purpose of inducing an internal cleansing of the colon and digestive tract

Core strength–the utilization of muscles designed to add structure and stabilization strength to the torso (i.e., abdominals, transverse abdominis, spinal erectors, obliques, hip flexors, etc.)

Detoxify–the removal of toxic substances from the body

Dietary fiber–any substance, generally of plant origin,

which is undigested on passage through the human alimentary tract, consists mostly of complex carbohydrates.

Dietician–an expert in food and nutrition. Dietitians help promote good health through proper eating. They also supervise the preparation and service of food, develop modified diets, participate in research, and educate individuals and groups on good nutritional habits.

Empty fat calories–calories consumed from food sources with a relatively high fat content proportionate to protein and carbohydrate having a low overall nutrient value

Energy storage–the storing of some form of energy that can be drawn upon at a later time to perform some useful operation

Exercise–bodily activity that develops and maintains physical fitness and overall health. It is often practiced to strengthen muscles and the cardiovascular system and to hone athletic skills. Frequent and regular physical exercise boosts the immune system and helps prevent diseases such as heart disease, cardiovascular disease, type 2 diabetes, and obesity.

Exercise physiology–a discipline involving the study of how exercise alters the structure and function of the human body

Fat–reserve energy stored in the form of lipids in adipose (tissue that contains fat storage cells) tissue

Flexor–a muscle whose contraction acts to bend a joint or limb

Formaldehyde–Formaldehyde-based solutions are used in the embalming process to disinfect and temporarily preserve human remains.

Free radicals–Free radicals are very unstable and react quickly with many other compounds, attempting to capture the needed electron to gain stability. Free radicals attack the nearest stable molecule, "robbing" it of its electron. When the "robbed" molecule loses its electron, it becomes a free radical itself, creating a chain reaction. Once the process has begun, it can cascade, finally resulting in the disruption of a living cell, causing damage to living tissues.

Functional training–a classification of exercise which involves training the body for the activities performed in daily life

Glucose transport–the means by which the bloodstream transports sugars through the circulatory system to the various systems for fuel (liver, muscles, pancreas, etc.)

Glycogen–functions as an immediate reserve source of available glucose for muscle cells

Heart-rate monitor–a device that allows a user to measure his or her heart rate in real time. It usually consists of two elements: a chest strap transmitter and a wrist receiver.

Herbs–a plant that is valued for qualities such as medicinal properties, flavor, scent, or the like

Hip flexors–a group of muscles that act to flex the femur onto the lumbo-pelvic complex

Hydration–the process of providing an adequate amount of water to body tissues

Hypertension–the disease or disorder of abnormally high blood pressure

Isolation exercise–exercise with a singular focus on a particular muscle or movement

Kinesiology–the science of human movement. It focuses on how the body functions and moves.

Lean mass–any human tissue not containing adipose tissue or means for lipid/fat storage (i.e., muscle tissue, organ tissue, etc.)

Leptin levels–the amount of protein hormones that plays a key role in regulating energy intake and energy expenditure. These processes include appetite and energy metabolism. Leptin is among the most important adipose originating hormones.

Lipids–fat-soluble molecules whose primary function is reserve energy storage and to provide cell structure

Macronutrient–nutrients needed in relatively large quantities (i.e. carbohydrates, fats, and proteins)

Maintenance–the process in which one adopts a sustainable process of nutrition and exercise with the purpose of maintaining current conditioning and body composition levels

Master trainer–A master trainer is a credentialed health and fitness professional who holds at least a Bachelor of Sciences degree, two industry recognized personal training certifications, and has a minimum of ten thousand session hours experience.

Mean composition ratio–the relation between balanced components for a given makeup (i.e., percentages protein, carbohydrate, and fat for meal composition) averaged

Metabolic rate–the overall rate at which the digestive and enzymatic processes in the body breakdown food components into usable energy

Metabolism–the process by which the human body breaks down food components into usable energy

Micronutrient–nutrients needed for life in small quantities (i.e., iron, cobalt, chromium, copper, iodine, manganese, selenium, zinc, and molybdenum)

Moderation–something which avoids excesses

Mono-unsaturated fat–foods containing monounsaturated fats lower LDL cholesterol, while possibly raising HDL cholesterol as well as providing some of the same cell protective benefits as polyunsaturated fats

Morbidly obese–a condition in which the natural energy reserve, stored in the fatty tissue of humans and other mammals, exceeds healthy limits

Nutrition program–a proficiently designed program for meal composition, timing, and energy density designed with a specific goal in mind

Nutritional data–data provided on commercially purchased food products detailing the composition and nutritional make up of the contents, or data made available on databases such as on the USDA Web site

Nutritional supplementation–a preparation intended to supply nutrients (such as vitamins, minerals, fatty acids, or amino acids) that are missing or not consumed in sufficient quantity in a person's diet

Nutritionist–a health specialist who devotes professional activity to food and nutritional science, preventive nutrition, diseases related to nutrient deficiencies, and the use of nutrient manipulation to enhance the clinical response to human diseases

Obliques–the abdominal muscles responsible for rotation of the trunk

Omega 3–a family of unsaturated fatty acids

Omega 6–a family of unsaturated fatty acids

Omega 9–a family of unsaturated fatty acids

Organic–foods produced according to certain production standards. It means they were grown without the use of conventional pesticides, artificial fertilizers, human waste, or sewage sludge and that they were processed without ionizing radiation or food additives

Osteoarthritis–a form of arthritis, affecting mainly older people, caused by chronic degeneration of the cartilage and synovial fluid of the joints, leading to pain and stiffness

Osteoporosis–a disease, occurring especially in women following menopause, in which the bones become extremely porous and are subject to fracture

Pancreatic response–the insulin hormone response by the pancreas induced by consumption of sugary or high-starch foods

Partially hydrogenated fat–a cooking fat or oil that has been infused with hydrogen molecules to increase shelf life and stability. These fats also pose potentially serious health complications.

Pectoral muscles (major)–a thick, fan-shaped muscle, situated at the upper front (anterior) of the chest wall. It makes up the bulk of the chest muscles in the male and lies under the breast in the female.

Personal training certification–a credential awarded to a health and fitness professional upon completion of an extensive academic and/or practical curriculum for the purpose of designing and implementing exercise programs and providing basic nutritional guidance

Phytonutrients–any substance of plant origin that provides nutrition

Plateau–a comparatively stable level in something that varies

Poly-unsaturated fat–polyunsaturated fat, along with monounsaturated fat are "beneficial fats." Polyunsaturated fat can be found mostly in some grain products, fish and sea food, and fish oil.

Postural assessment–an assessment conducted by a health and fitness professional to determine any structural misalignments, strength imbalances, and skeletal abnormalities

Postural maladies–abnormal condition in the musculo-skeletal system leading to movement and range of motion distortions

Postural misalignment–the condition in which the joint connecting points for two bones has been compromised leading to motion abnormalities

Professional fitness assessment–the initial and or follow-up assessment by a certified health and fitness professional to determine the physical fitness level of a particular individual. Typical assessment might include: cardio-respiratory efficiency, upper-body peripheral strength, lower-body peripheral strength, core strength, flexibility, and balance.

Protein–one of three major classes of food or source of food energy (four <u>kcal</u>/gram) abundant in animal-derived foods (*i.e., meat*) and some vegetables, such as legumes

Saturated fat–a fat or oil, from either animal or vegetable sources, containing a high proportion of saturated fatty acids, will typically be solid at room temperature; a diet high in saturated rather than unsaturated fats is thought to contribute to higher levels of cholesterol in the blood.

Shoulder girdle stabilizers–muscle complex in the shoulder girdle complex responsible for maintaining structural integrity where the upper arm connects to the torso

Sodium–common mineral used in the preservation process of many food products including meats and dairy products to increase shelf life and stability. High levels of consumption have been shown to increase risk for cardiovascular disease as well as compromise the body's natural hydro-regulatory system.

Spinal erectors–erectorspinae muscles found along the spinal column whose purpose is to facilitate disc movement and maintain alignment

Spot training–the false belief that exercising a specific muscle will result in a decrease in the amount of fat in the area surrounding that muscle. A common example of this is focusing on abdominal exercises in an effort to lose weight in or around one's stomach.

Stability ball–ball constructed of elastic soft PVC with a diameter of around thirty-five to eighty-five cm (fourteen to thirty-four inches). It is used in physical therapy and exercise. Also known by a number of different names, including **balance ball, birth ball, body ball, exercise ball, fitness ball, gym ball, physioball, Pilates ball, sports ball, Swiss ball, Swedish ball, therapy ball**, or **yoga ball**

Strength imbalance–an irregular shortening of one muscle and lengthening of another for a given range of motion, creating postural imbalances and maladies as well as compromising joint integrity

Strength training–the use of resistance to build the strength, anaerobic endurance, and size of skeletal muscles. When properly performed, strength training can provide significant functional benefits and improvement in overall health and well-being including increased bone, muscle, tendon, and ligament strength and toughness, improved joint function, reduced potential for injury, improved cardiac function, and elevated good cholesterol.

Subcutaneous fat–fat that is found just beneath the skin

Sustainability–the ability to maintain (*something*) or to keep it in existence

Trans fat–common name for a type of unsaturated fat. Trans fats may be monunsaturated or polyunsaturated. Most trans fats consumed today are industrially created by partially hydrogenating plant oils.

Type 2 diabetes–(formerly called non-insulin-dependent diabetes mellitus NIDDM, or adult-onset diabetes) a metabolic disorder that is primarily characterized by insulin resistance, relative insulin deficiency, and hyperglycemia (high blood sugar)

Uni-planar machine–exercise machine that travels in a singular/set plane of motion (rarely suitable for optimal natural movement strengthening)

Upper body strength assessment–a structured assessment (typically a push/pull assessment) conducted by a health and fitness professional with the purpose of determining upper body strength capabilities of a client

Visceral fat–(also known as organ fat) fat that is packed in between internal organs

Weight-loss supplement–a nutritional supplement designed to aid in weight loss and metabolic efficiency. Many of these supplements have little to no documented efficacy often with serious adverse side effects and complications.

YOUR BODY, YOUR LIFE, YOURSELF JOURNAL

Copy the following pages as needed

WORKOUT LOG

Day of Week: M - T - W - Th - F - Sa - Su
Date @ Time: _____

CARDIOVASCULAR WORKOUT   Time Spent: _____

EXERCISE	Time	Distance	Average HR or Intensity Level	Calories Burned	Comments

STRENGTH TRAINING   { ❑ Upper Body ❑ Lower Body ❑ Abs }   Time Spent: _____

EXERCISE		1st Set	2nd Set	3rd Set	4th Set	5th Set	6th Set	Comments
	REP							
	WT							
	REP							
	WT							
	REP							
	WT							
	REP							
	WT							
	REP							
	WT							
	REP							
	WT							
	REP							
	WT							
	REP							
	WT							

STRETCHING   Time Spent: _____

EXERCISE	Duration	Comments

Day of Week: M - T - W - Th - F - Sa - Su
Date: _____

NUTRITION LOG

DAILY GOAL	Calories	Protein (gr)	Carbs (gr)	Fat (gr)	Water (oz)	Comments

ACTUAL CONSUMPTION

FOODS	Calories	Protein (gr)	Carbs (gr)	Fat (gr)	Water (oz)	Comments
AM/PM MEAL ONE						
AM/PM MEAL TWO						
AM/PM MEAL THREE						
AM/PM MEAL FOUR						
AM/PM MEAL FIVE						
AM/PM MEAL SIX						
TOTAL						

SUPPLEMENTS

WORKOUT LOG

Day of Week: M - T - W - Th - F - Sa - Su
Date @ Time: _____

CARDIOVASCULAR WORKOUT   Time Spent: _____

EXERCISE	Time	Distance	Average HR or Intensity Level	Calories Burned	Comments

STRENGTH TRAINING   { ❑ Upper Body ❑ Lower Body ❑ Abs }   Time Spent: _____

EXERCISE		1st Set	2nd Set	3rd Set	4th Set	5th Set	6th Set	Comments
	REP							
	WT							
	REP							
	WT							
	REP							
	WT							
	REP							
	WT							
	REP							
	WT							
	REP							
	WT							
	REP							
	WT							
	REP							
	WT							

STRETCHING   Time Spent: _____

EXERCISE	Duration	Comments

Day of Week: M - T - W - Th - F - Sa - Su
Date: _____

NUTRITION LOG

DAILY GOAL	Calories	Protein (gr)	Carbs (gr)	Fat (gr)	Water (oz)	Comments

ACTUAL CONSUMPTION

FOODS	Calories	Protein (gr)	Carbs (gr)	Fat (gr)	Water (oz)	Comments
AM PM MEAL ONE						
AM PM MEAL TWO						
AM PM MEAL THREE						
AM PM MEAL FOUR						
AM PM MEAL FIVE						
AM PM MEAL SIX						
TOTAL						

SUPPLEMENTS

_____

_____

WORKOUT LOG

Day of Week: M - T - W - Th - F - Sa - S
Date @ Time: _____

CARDIOVASCULAR WORKOUT   Time Spent: _____

EXERCISE	Time	Distance	Average HR or Intensity Level	Calories Burned	Comments

STRENGTH TRAINING   { ☐ Upper Body ☐ Lower Body ☐ Abs }   Time Spent: _____

EXERCISE		1st Set	2nd Set	3rd Set	4th Set	5th Set	6th Set	Comments
	REP							
	WT							
	REP							
	WT							
	REP							
	WT							
	REP							
	WT							
	REP							
	WT							
	REP							
	WT							
	REP							
	WT							
	REP							
	WT							

STRETCHING   Time Spent: _____

EXERCISE	Duration	Comments

Day of Week: M - T - W - Th - F - Sa - Su
Date: _____

NUTRITION LOG

DAILY GOAL	Calories	Protein (gr)	Carbs (gr)	Fat (gr)	Water (oz)	Comments

ACTUAL CONSUMPTION

FOODS	Calories	Protein (gr)	Carbs (gr)	Fat (gr)	Water (oz)	Comments
AM PM MEAL ONE						
AM PM MEAL TWO						
AM PM MEAL THREE						
AM PM MEAL FOUR						
AM PM MEAL FIVE						
AM PM MEAL SIX						
TOTAL						

SUPPLEMENTS

WORKOUT LOG

Day of Week: M - T - W - Th - F - Sa - Su
Date @ Time: _____

CARDIOVASCULAR WORKOUT   Time Spent: _____

EXERCISE	Time	Distance	Average HR or Intensity Level	Calories Burned	Comments

STRENGTH TRAINING { ❑ Upper Body ❑ Lower Body ❑ Abs }   Time Spent: _____

EXERCISE		1st Set	2nd Set	3rd Set	4th Set	5th Set	6th Set	Comments
	REP							
	WT							
	REP							
	WT							
	REP							
	WT							
	REP							
	WT							
	REP							
	WT							
	REP							
	WT							
	REP							
	WT							
	REP							
	WT							

STRETCHING   Time Spent: _____

EXERCISE	Duration	Comments

Day of Week: M - T - W - Th - F - Sa - Su
Date: _____

NUTRITION LOG

DAILY GOAL	Calories	Protein (gr)	Carbs (gr)	Fat (gr)	Water (oz)	Comments

ACTUAL CONSUMPTION

FOODS	Calories	Protein (gr)	Carbs (gr)	Fat (gr)	Water (oz)	Comments
AM/PM MEAL ONE						
AM/PM MEAL TWO						
AM/PM MEAL THREE						
AM/PM MEAL FOUR						
AM/PM MEAL FIVE						
AM/PM MEAL SIX						
TOTAL						

SUPPLEMENTS

_____

_____

WORKOUT LOG

Day of Week: M - T - W - Th - F - Sa - Su
Date @ Time: _____

CARDIOVASCULAR WORKOUT   Time Spent: _____

EXERCISE	Time	Distance	Average HR or Intensity Level	Calories Burned	Comments

STRENGTH TRAINING   { ❏ Upper Body ❏ Lower Body ❏ Abs }   Time Spent: _____

EXERCISE		1st Set	2nd Set	3rd Set	4th Set	5th Set	6th Set	Comments
	REP							
	WT							
	REP							
	WT							
	REP							
	WT							
	REP							
	WT							
	REP							
	WT							
	REP							
	WT							
	REP							
	WT							
	REP							
	WT							

STRETCHING   Time Spent: _____

EXERCISE	Duration	Comments

Day of Week: M - T - W - Th - F - Sa - Su
Date: _____

NUTRITION LOG

DAILY GOAL	Calories	Protein (gr)	Carbs (gr)	Fat (gr)	Water (oz)	Comments

ACTUAL CONSUMPTION

FOODS	Calories	Protein (gr)	Carbs (gr)	Fat (gr)	Water (oz)	Comments
AM PM — MEAL ONE						
AM PM — MEAL TWO						
AM PM — MEAL THREE						
AM PM — MEAL FOUR						
AM PM — MEAL FIVE						
AM PM — MEAL SIX						
TOTAL						

SUPPLEMENTS

_____

_____

WORKOUT LOG

Day of Week: M - T - W - Th - F - Sa - Su
Date @ Time: _____

CARDIOVASCULAR WORKOUT   Time Spent: _____

EXERCISE	Time	Distance	Average HR or Intensity Level	Calories Burned	Comments

STRENGTH TRAINING   { ☐ Upper Body ☐ Lower Body ☐ Abs } Time Spent: _____

EXERCISE		1st Set	2nd Set	3rd Set	4th Set	5th Set	6th Set	Comments
	REP							
	WT							
	REP							
	WT							
	REP							
	WT							
	REP							
	WT							
	REP							
	WT							
	REP							
	WT							
	REP							
	WT							
	REP							
	WT							

STRETCHING   Time Spent: _____

EXERCISE	Duration	Comments

Day of Week: M - T - W - Th - F - Sa - Su
Date: _____

NUTRITION LOG

DAILY GOAL	Calories	Protein (gr)	Carbs (gr)	Fat (gr)	Water (oz)	Comments

ACTUAL CONSUMPTION

FOODS		Calories	Protein (gr)	Carbs (gr)	Fat (gr)	Water (oz)	Comments
MEAL ONE	AM/PM						
MEAL TWO	AM/PM						
MEAL THREE	AM/PM						
MEAL FOUR	AM/PM						
MEAL FIVE	AM/PM						
MEAL SIX	AM/PM						
TOTAL							

SUPPLEMENTS

_____

_____

WORKOUT LOG

Day of Week: M - T - W - Th - F - Sa - Su
Date @ Time: _____

CARDIOVASCULAR WORKOUT   Time Spent: _____

EXERCISE	Time	Distance	Average HR or Intensity Level	Calories Burned	Comments

STRENGTH TRAINING   { ❑ Upper Body ❑ Lower Body ❑ Abs }   Time Spent: _____

EXERCISE		1st Set	2nd Set	3rd Set	4th Set	5th Set	6th Set	Comments
	REP							
	WT							
	REP							
	WT							
	REP							
	WT							
	REP							
	WT							
	REP							
	WT							
	REP							
	WT							
	REP							
	WT							
	REP							
	WT							

STRETCHING   Time Spent: _____

EXERCISE	Duration	Comments

Day of Week: M - T - W - Th - F - Sa - Su
Date: _____

NUTRITION LOG

DAILY GOAL	Calories	Protein (gr)	Carbs (gr)	Fat (gr)	Water (oz)	Comments

ACTUAL CONSUMPTION

FOODS	Calories	Protein (gr)	Carbs (gr)	Fat (gr)	Water (oz)	Comments
AM/PM MEAL ONE						
AM/PM MEAL TWO						
AM/PM MEAL THREE						
AM/PM MEAL FOUR						
AM/PM MEAL FIVE						
AM/PM MEAL SIX						
TOTAL						

SUPPLEMENTS

WORKOUT LOG

CARDIOVASCULAR WORKOUT   Time Spent: _____

EXERCISE	Time	Distance	Average HR or Intensity Level	Calories Burned	Comments

STRENGTH TRAINING   { ❑ Upper Body ❑ Lower Body ❑ Abs }   Time Spent: _____

EXERCISE		1st Set	2nd Set	3rd Set	4th Set	5th Set	6th Set	Comments
	REP							
	WT							
	REP							
	WT							
	REP							
	WT							
	REP							
	WT							
	REP							
	WT							
	REP							
	WT							
	REP							
	WT							
	REP							
	WT							

STRETCHING   Time Spent: _____

EXERCISE	Duration	Comments

Day of Week: M - T - W - Th - F - Sa - Su
Date: _____

NUTRITION LOG

DAILY GOAL	Calories	Protein (gr)	Carbs (gr)	Fat (gr)	Water (oz)	Comments

ACTUAL CONSUMPTION

FOODS	Calories	Protein (gr)	Carbs (gr)	Fat (gr)	Water (oz)	Comments
AM/PM MEAL ONE						
AM/PM MEAL TWO						
AM/PM MEAL THREE						
AM/PM MEAL FOUR						
AM/PM MEAL FIVE						
AM/PM MEAL SIX						
TOTAL						

SUPPLEMENTS

_____

_____

WORKOUT LOG

Day of Week: M - T - W - Th - F - Sa - Su
Date @ Time: _____

CARDIOVASCULAR WORKOUT   Time Spent: _____

EXERCISE	Time	Distance	Average HR or Intensity Level	Calories Burned	Comments

STRENGTH TRAINING   { ❑ Upper Body ❑ Lower Body ❑ Abs }   Time Spent: _____

EXERCISE		1st Set	2nd Set	3rd Set	4th Set	5th Set	6th Set	Comments
	REP							
	WT							
	REP							
	WT							
	REP							
	WT							
	REP							
	WT							
	REP							
	WT							
	REP							
	WT							
	REP							
	WT							
	REP							
	WT							

STRETCHING   Time Spent: _____

EXERCISE	Duration	Comments

Day of Week: M - T - W - Th - F - Sa - Su
Date: _____

NUTRITION LOG

DAILY GOAL	Calories	Protein (gr)	Carbs (gr)	Fat (gr)	Water (oz)	Comments

ACTUAL CONSUMPTION

FOODS	Calories	Protein (gr)	Carbs (gr)	Fat (gr)	Water (oz)	Comments
AM PM MEAL ONE						
AM PM MEAL TWO						
AM PM MEAL THREE						
AM PM MEAL FOUR						
AM PM MEAL FIVE						
AM PM MEAL SIX						
TOTAL						

SUPPLEMENTS

_____

_____

WORKOUT LOG

Day of Week: M - T - W - Th - F - Sa - Su
Date @ Time: _____

CARDIOVASCULAR WORKOUT   Time Spent: _____

EXERCISE	Time	Distance	Average HR or Intensity Level	Calories Burned	Comments

STRENGTH TRAINING   { ❑ Upper Body ❑ Lower Body ❑ Abs }   Time Spent: _____

EXERCISE		1st Set	2nd Set	3rd Set	4th Set	5th Set	6th Set	Comments
	REP							
	WT							
	REP							
	WT							
	REP							
	WT							
	REP							
	WT							
	REP							
	WT							
	REP							
	WT							
	REP							
	WT							
	REP							
	WT							

STRETCHING   Time Spent: _____

EXERCISE	Duration	Comments

Day of Week: M - T - W - Th - F - Sa - Su
Date: _____

NUTRITION LOG

DAILY GOAL	Calories	Protein (gr)	Carbs (gr)	Fat (gr)	Water (oz)	Comments

ACTUAL CONSUMPTION

FOODS		Calories	Protein (gr)	Carbs (gr)	Fat (gr)	Water (oz)	Comments
MEAL ONE	AM PM						
MEAL TWO	AM PM						
MEAL THREE	AM PM						
MEAL FOUR	AM PM						
MEAL FIVE	AM PM						
MEAL SIX	AM PM						
TOTAL							

SUPPLEMENTS

WORKOUT LOG

Day of Week: M - T - W - Th - F - Sa - Su
Date @ Time: _____

CARDIOVASCULAR WORKOUT   Time Spent: _____

EXERCISE	Time	Distance	Average HR or Intensity Level	Calories Burned	Comments

STRENGTH TRAINING   { ❑ Upper Body ❑ Lower Body ❑ Abs }   Time Spent: _____

EXERCISE		1st Set	2nd Set	3rd Set	4th Set	5th Set	6th Set	Comments
	REP							
	WT							
	REP							
	WT							
	REP							
	WT							
	REP							
	WT							
	REP							
	WT							
	REP							
	WT							
	REP							
	WT							
	REP							
	WT							

STRETCHING   Time Spent: _____

EXERCISE	Duration	Comments

Day of Week: M - T - W - Th - F - Sa - Su
Date: _____

NUTRITION LOG

DAILY GOAL	Calories	Protein (gr)	Carbs (gr)	Fat (gr)	Water (oz)	Comments

ACTUAL CONSUMPTION

FOODS	Calories	Protein (gr)	Carbs (gr)	Fat (gr)	Water (oz)	Comments
AM PM MEAL ONE						
AM PM MEAL TWO						
AM PM MEAL THREE						
AM PM MEAL FOUR						
AM PM MEAL FIVE						
AM PM MEAL SIX						
TOTAL						

SUPPLEMENTS

_____

_____

WORKOUT LOG

Day of Week: M - T - W - Th - F - Sa - Su
Date @ Time: _____

CARDIOVASCULAR WORKOUT   Time Spent: _____

EXERCISE	Time	Distance	Average HR or Intensity Level	Calories Burned	Comments

STRENGTH TRAINING   { ❑ Upper Body ❑ Lower Body ❑ Abs } Time Spent: _____

EXERCISE		1ˢᵗ Set	2ⁿᵈ Set	3ʳᵈ Set	4ᵗʰ Set	5ᵗʰ Set	6ᵗʰ Set	Comments
	REP							
	WT							
	REP							
	WT							
	REP							
	WT							
	REP							
	WT							
	REP							
	WT							
	REP							
	WT							
	REP							
	WT							
	REP							
	WT							

STRETCHING   Time Spent: _____

EXERCISE	Duration	Comments

Day of Week: M - T - W - Th - F - Sa - Su
Date: _____

NUTRITION LOG

DAILY GOAL	Calories	Protein (gr)	Carbs (gr)	Fat (gr)	Water (oz)	Comments

ACTUAL CONSUMPTION

FOODS	Calories	Protein (gr)	Carbs (gr)	Fat (gr)	Water (oz)	Comments
AM PM MEAL ONE						
AM PM MEAL TWO						
AM PM MEAL THREE						
AM PM MEAL FOUR						
AM PM MEAL FIVE						
AM PM MEAL SIX						
TOTAL						

SUPPLEMENTS

_____

_____

WORKOUT LOG

Day of Week: M - T - W - Th - F - Sa - Su
Date @ Time: _____

CARDIOVASCULAR WORKOUT   Time Spent: _____

EXERCISE	Time	Distance	Average HR or Intensity Level	Calories Burned	Comments

STRENGTH TRAINING { ❑ Upper Body ❑ Lower Body ❑ Abs } Time Spent: _____

EXERCISE		1st Set	2nd Set	3rd Set	4th Set	5th Set	6th Set	Comments
	REP							
	WT							
	REP							
	WT							
	REP							
	WT							
	REP							
	WT							
	REP							
	WT							
	REP							
	WT							
	REP							
	WT							
	REP							
	WT							

STRETCHING   Time Spent: _____

EXERCISE	Duration	Comments

Day of Week: M - T - W - Th - F - Sa - Su

Date: _____

NUTRITION LOG

DAILY GOAL	Calories	Protein (gr)	Carbs (gr)	Fat (gr)	Water (oz)	Comments

ACTUAL CONSUMPTION

FOODS	Calories	Protein (gr)	Carbs (gr)	Fat (gr)	Water (oz)	Comments
AM/PM MEAL ONE						
AM/PM MEAL TWO						
AM/PM MEAL THREE						
AM/PM MEAL FOUR						
AM/PM MEAL FIVE						
AM/PM MEAL SIX						
TOTAL						

SUPPLEMENTS

_____

_____

WORKOUT LOG

Day of Week: M - T - W - Th - F - Sa - Su
Date @ Time: _____

CARDIOVASCULAR WORKOUT   Time Spent: _____

EXERCISE	Time	Distance	Average HR or Intensity Level	Calories Burned	Comments

STRENGTH TRAINING { ❑ Upper Body ❑ Lower Body ❑ Abs } Time Spent: _____

EXERCISE		1st Set	2nd Set	3rd Set	4th Set	5th Set	6th Set	Comments
	REP							
	WT							
	REP							
	WT							
	REP							
	WT							
	REP							
	WT							
	REP							
	WT							
	REP							
	WT							
	REP							
	WT							
	REP							
	WT							

STRETCHING   Time Spent: _____

EXERCISE	Duration	Comments

Day of Week: M - T - W - Th - F - Sa - Su
Date: _____

NUTRITION LOG

DAILY GOAL	Calories	Protein (gr)	Carbs (gr)	Fat (gr)	Water (oz)	Comments

ACTUAL CONSUMPTION

FOODS	Calories	Protein (gr)	Carbs (gr)	Fat (gr)	Water (oz)	Comments
AM PM MEAL ONE						
AM PM MEAL TWO						
AM PM MEAL THREE						
AM PM MEAL FOUR						
AM PM MEAL FIVE						
AM PM MEAL SIX						
TOTAL						

SUPPLEMENTS

WORKOUT LOG

Day of Week: M - T - W - Th - F - Sa - Su
Date @ Time: _____

CARDIOVASCULAR WORKOUT   Time Spent: _____

EXERCISE	Time	Distance	Average HR or Intensity Level	Calories Burned	Comments

STRENGTH TRAINING   { ❑ Upper Body ❑ Lower Body ❑ Abs }   Time Spent: _____

EXERCISE		1st Set	2nd Set	3rd Set	4th Set	5th Set	6th Set	Comments
	REP							
	WT							
	REP							
	WT							
	REP							
	WT							
	REP							
	WT							
	REP							
	WT							
	REP							
	WT							
	REP							
	WT							
	REP							
	WT							

STRETCHING   Time Spent: _____

EXERCISE	Duration	Comments

Day of Week: M - T - W - Th - F - Sa - Su
Date: _____

NUTRITION LOG

DAILY GOAL	Calories	Protein (gr)	Carbs (gr)	Fat (gr)	Water (oz)	Comments

ACTUAL CONSUMPTION

FOODS	Calories	Protein (gr)	Carbs (gr)	Fat (gr)	Water (oz)	Comments
AM PM — MEAL ONE						
AM PM — MEAL TWO						
AM PM — MEAL THREE						
AM PM — MEAL FOUR						
AM PM — MEAL FIVE						
MEAL SIX						
TOTAL						

SUPPLEMENTS

WORKOUT LOG

Day of Week: M - T - W - Th - F - Sa - Su
Date @ Time: _____

CARDIOVASCULAR WORKOUT   Time Spent: _____

EXERCISE	Time	Distance	Average HR or Intensity Level	Calories Burned	Comments

STRENGTH TRAINING { ❑ Upper Body ❑ Lower Body ❑ Abs } Time Spent: _____

EXERCISE		1st Set	2nd Set	3rd Set	4th Set	5th Set	6th Set	Comments
	REP							
	WT							
	REP							
	WT							
	REP							
	WT							
	REP							
	WT							
	REP							
	WT							
	REP							
	WT							
	REP							
	WT							
	REP							
	WT							

STRETCHING   Time Spent: _____

EXERCISE	Duration	Comments

Day of Week: M - T - W - Th - F - Sa - Su
Date: _____

NUTRITION LOG

DAILY GOAL	Calories	Protein (gr)	Carbs (gr)	Fat (gr)	Water (oz)	Comments

ACTUAL CONSUMPTION

FOODS	Calories	Protein (gr)	Carbs (gr)	Fat (gr)	Water (oz)	Comments
AM/PM MEAL ONE						
AM/PM MEAL TWO						
AM/PM MEAL THREE						
AM/PM MEAL FOUR						
AM/PM MEAL FIVE						
AM/PM MEAL SIX						
TOTAL						

SUPPLEMENTS

_____

_____

WORKOUT LOG

CARDIOVASCULAR WORKOUT   Time Spent: _____

EXERCISE	Time	Distance	Average HR or Intensity Level	Calories Burned	Comments

STRENGTH TRAINING { ❑ Upper Body ❑ Lower Body ❑ Abs } Time Spent: _____

EXERCISE		1st Set	2nd Set	3rd Set	4th Set	5th Set	6th Set	Comments
	REP							
	WT							
	REP							
	WT							
	REP							
	WT							
	REP							
	WT							
	REP							
	WT							
	REP							
	WT							
	REP							
	WT							
	REP							
	WT							

STRETCHING   Time Spent: _____

EXERCISE	Duration	Comments

Day of Week: M - T - W - Th - F - Sa - Su
Date: _____

NUTRITION LOG

DAILY GOAL	Calories	Protein (gr)	Carbs (gr)	Fat (gr)	Water (oz)	Comments

ACTUAL CONSUMPTION

FOODS	Calories	Protein (gr)	Carbs (gr)	Fat (gr)	Water (oz)	Comments
AM/PM MEAL ONE						
AM/PM MEAL TWO						
AM/PM MEAL THREE						
AM/PM MEAL FOUR						
AM/PM MEAL FIVE						
AM/PM MEAL SIX						
TOTAL						

SUPPLEMENTS

WORKOUT LOG

Day of Week: M - T - W - Th - F - Sa - Su
Date @ Time: _____

CARDIOVASCULAR WORKOUT   Time Spent: _____

EXERCISE	Time	Distance	Average HR or Intensity Level	Calories Burned	Comments

STRENGTH TRAINING   { ☐ Upper Body ☐ Lower Body ☐ Abs }   Time Spent: _____

EXERCISE		1st Set	2nd Set	3rd Set	4th Set	5th Set	6th Set	Comments
	REP							
	WT							
	REP							
	WT							
	REP							
	WT							
	REP							
	WT							
	REP							
	WT							
	REP							
	WT							
	REP							
	WT							
	REP							
	WT							

STRETCHING   Time Spent: _____

EXERCISE	Duration	Comments

Day of Week: M - T - W - Th - F - Sa - Su
Date: _____

NUTRITION LOG

DAILY GOAL	Calories	Protein (gr)	Carbs (gr)	Fat (gr)	Water (oz)	Comments

ACTUAL CONSUMPTION

FOODS		Calories	Protein (gr)	Carbs (gr)	Fat (gr)	Water (oz)	Comments
MEAL ONE	AM PM						
MEAL TWO	AM PM						
MEAL THREE	AM PM						
MEAL FOUR	AM PM						
MEAL FIVE	AM PM						
MEAL SIX	AM PM						
TOTAL							

SUPPLEMENTS

_____

_____

WORKOUT LOG

CARDIOVASCULAR WORKOUT   Time Spent: _____

EXERCISE	Time	Distance	Average HR or Intensity Level	Calories Burned	Comments

STRENGTH TRAINING { ❑ Upper Body ❑ Lower Body ❑ Abs } Time Spent: _____

EXERCISE		1st Set	2nd Set	3rd Set	4th Set	5th Set	6th Set	Comments
	REP							
	WT							
	REP							
	WT							
	REP							
	WT							
	REP							
	WT							
	REP							
	WT							
	REP							
	WT							
	REP							
	WT							
	REP							
	WT							

STRETCHING   Time Spent: _____

EXERCISE	Duration	Comments

Day of Week: M - T - W - Th - F - Sa - Su
Date: _____

NUTRITION LOG

DAILY GOAL	Calories	Protein (gr)	Carbs (gr)	Fat (gr)	Water (oz)	Comments

ACTUAL CONSUMPTION

FOODS	Calories	Protein (gr)	Carbs (gr)	Fat (gr)	Water (oz)	Comments
AM PM MEAL ONE						
AM PM MEAL TWO						
AM PM MEAL THREE						
AM PM MEAL FOUR						
AM PM MEAL FIVE						
AM PM MEAL SIX						
TOTAL						

SUPPLEMENTS

_____

_____

WORKOUT LOG

Day of Week: M - T - W - Th - F - Sa - Su
Date @ Time: _____

CARDIOVASCULAR WORKOUT   Time Spent: _____

EXERCISE	Time	Distance	Average HR or Intensity Level	Calories Burned	Comments

STRENGTH TRAINING   { ❑ Upper Body ❑ Lower Body ❑ Abs }   Time Spent: _____

EXERCISE		1st Set	2nd Set	3rd Set	4th Set	5th Set	6th Set	Comments
	REP							
	WT							
	REP							
	WT							
	REP							
	WT							
	REP							
	WT							
	REP							
	WT							
	REP							
	WT							
	REP							
	WT							
	REP							
	WT							

STRETCHING   Time Spent: _____

EXERCISE	Duration	Comments

Day of Week: M - T - W - Th - F - Sa - Su
Date: _____

NUTRITION LOG

DAILY GOAL	Calories	Protein (gr)	Carbs (gr)	Fat (gr)	Water (oz)	Comments

ACTUAL CONSUMPTION

FOODS	Calories	Protein (gr)	Carbs (gr)	Fat (gr)	Water (oz)	Comments
AM PM MEAL ONE						
AM PM MEAL TWO						
AM PM MEAL THREE						
AM PM MEAL FOUR						
AM PM MEAL FIVE						
AM PM MEAL SIX						
TOTAL						

SUPPLEMENTS

WORKOUT LOG

Day of Week: M - T - W - Th - F - Sa - Su
Date @ Time: _____

CARDIOVASCULAR WORKOUT   Time Spent: _____

EXERCISE	Time	Distance	Average HR or Intensity Level	Calories Burned	Comments

STRENGTH TRAINING   { ❑ Upper Body ❑ Lower Body ❑ Abs }   Time Spent: _____

EXERCISE		1st Set	2nd Set	3rd Set	4th Set	5th Set	6th Set	Comments
	REP							
	WT							
	REP							
	WT							
	REP							
	WT							
	REP							
	WT							
	REP							
	WT							
	REP							
	WT							
	REP							
	WT							
	REP							
	WT							

STRETCHING   Time Spent: _____

EXERCISE	Duration	Comments

Day of Week: M - T - W - Th - F - Sa - Su
Date: _____

NUTRITION LOG

DAILY GOAL	Calories	Protein (gr)	Carbs (gr)	Fat (gr)	Water (oz)	Comments

ACTUAL CONSUMPTION

FOODS	Calories	Protein (gr)	Carbs (gr)	Fat (gr)	Water (oz)	Comments
AM/PM MEAL ONE						
AM/PM MEAL TWO						
AM/PM MEAL THREE						
AM/PM MEAL FOUR						
AM/PM MEAL FIVE						
AM/PM MEAL SIX						
TOTAL						

SUPPLEMENTS

WORKOUT LOG

Day of Week: M · T · W · Th · F · Sa · Su
Date @ Time: _____

CARDIOVASCULAR WORKOUT   Time Spent: _____

EXERCISE	Time	Distance	Average HR or Intensity Level	Calories Burned	Comments

STRENGTH TRAINING { ❑ Upper Body ❑ Lower Body ❑ Abs } Time Spent: _____

EXERCISE		1st Set	2nd Set	3rd Set	4th Set	5th Set	6th Set	Comments
	REP							
	WT							
	REP							
	WT							
	REP							
	WT							
	REP							
	WT							
	REP							
	WT							
	REP							
	WT							
	REP							
	WT							
	REP							
	WT							

STRETCHING   Time Spent: _____

EXERCISE	Duration	Comments

Day of Week: M - T - W - Th - F - Sa - Su
Date: _____

NUTRITION LOG

DAILY GOAL	Calories	Protein (gr)	Carbs (gr)	Fat (gr)	Water (oz)	Comments

ACTUAL CONSUMPTION

FOODS	Calories	Protein (gr)	Carbs (gr)	Fat (gr)	Water (oz)	Comments
AM PM MEAL ONE						
AM PM MEAL TWO						
AM PM MEAL THREE						
AM PM MEAL FOUR						
AM PM MEAL FIVE						
AM PM MEAL SIX						
TOTAL						

SUPPLEMENTS

_____

_____

WORKOUT LOG

Day of Week: M - T - W - Th - F - Sa - Su

Date @ Time: _____

CARDIOVASCULAR WORKOUT   Time Spent: _____

EXERCISE	Time	Distance	Average HR or Intensity Level	Calories Burned	Comments

STRENGTH TRAINING { ❑ Upper Body ❑ Lower Body ❑ Abs } Time Spent: _____

EXERCISE		1st Set	2nd Set	3rd Set	4th Set	5th Set	6th Set	Comments
	REP							
	WT							
	REP							
	WT							
	REP							
	WT							
	REP							
	WT							
	REP							
	WT							
	REP							
	WT							
	REP							
	WT							
	REP							
	WT							

STRETCHING   Time Spent: _____

EXERCISE	Duration	Comments

Day of Week: M - T - W - Th - F - Sa - Su
Date: _____

NUTRITION LOG

DAILY GOAL	Calories	Protein (gr)	Carbs (gr)	Fat (gr)	Water (oz)	Comments

ACTUAL CONSUMPTION

FOODS	Calories	Protein (gr)	Carbs (gr)	Fat (gr)	Water (oz)	Comments
AM PM — MEAL ONE						
AM PM — MEAL TWO						
AM PM — MEAL THREE						
AM PM — MEAL FOUR						
AM PM — MEAL FIVE						
AM PM — MEAL SIX						
TOTAL						

SUPPLEMENTS

WORKOUT LOG

Day of Week: M - T - W - Th - F - Sa - Su
Date @ Time: _____

CARDIOVASCULAR WORKOUT   Time Spent: _____

EXERCISE	Time	Distance	Average HR or Intensity Level	Calories Burned	Comments

STRENGTH TRAINING   { ❑ Upper Body ❑ Lower Body ❑ Abs }   Time Spent: _____

EXERCISE		1st Set	2nd Set	3rd Set	4th Set	5th Set	6th Set	Comments
	REP							
	WT							
	REP							
	WT							
	REP							
	WT							
	REP							
	WT							
	REP							
	WT							
	REP							
	WT							
	REP							
	WT							
	REP							
	WT							

STRETCHING   Time Spent: _____

EXERCISE	Duration	Comments

Day of Week: M - T - W - Th - F - Sa - Su
Date: _____

NUTRITION LOG

	Calories	Protein (gr)	Carbs (gr)	Fat (gr)	Water (oz)	Comments
DAILY GOAL						

ACTUAL CONSUMPTION

FOODS	Calories	Protein (gr)	Carbs (gr)	Fat (gr)	Water (oz)	Comments
AM PM MEAL ONE						
AM PM MEAL TWO						
AM PM MEAL THREE						
AM PM MEAL FOUR						
AM PM MEAL FIVE						
AM PM MEAL SIX						
TOTAL						

SUPPLEMENTS

WORKOUT LOG

Day of Week: M - T - W - Th - F - Sa - Su
Date @ Time: _____

CARDIOVASCULAR WORKOUT   Time Spent: _____

EXERCISE	Time	Distance	Average HR or Intensity Level	Calories Burned	Comments

STRENGTH TRAINING { ❑ Upper Body ❑ Lower Body ❑ Abs } Time Spent: _____

EXERCISE		1st Set	2nd Set	3rd Set	4th Set	5th Set	6th Set	Comments
	REP							
	WT							
	REP							
	WT							
	REP							
	WT							
	REP							
	WT							
	REP							
	WT							
	REP							
	WT							
	REP							
	WT							
	REP							
	WT							

STRETCHING   Time Spent: _____

EXERCISE	Duration	Comments

Day of Week: M - T - W - Th - F - Sa - Su

Date: _____

NUTRITION LOG

DAILY GOAL	Calories	Protein (gr)	Carbs (gr)	Fat (gr)	Water (oz)	Comments

ACTUAL CONSUMPTION

FOODS	Calories	Protein (gr)	Carbs (gr)	Fat (gr)	Water (oz)	Comments
MEAL ONE AM PM						
MEAL TWO AM PM						
MEAL THREE AM PM						
MEAL FOUR AM PM						
MEAL FIVE AM PM						
MEAL SIX AM PM						
TOTAL						

SUPPLEMENTS

_____

_____

WORKOUT LOG

Day of Week: M - T - W - Th - F - Sa - Su
Date @ Time: _____

CARDIOVASCULAR WORKOUT   Time Spent: _____

EXERCISE	Time	Distance	Average HR or Intensity Level	Calories Burned	Comments

STRENGTH TRAINING { ☐ Upper Body ☐ Lower Body ☐ Abs } Time Spent: _____

EXERCISE		1st Set	2nd Set	3rd Set	4th Set	5th Set	6th Set	Comments
	REP							
	WT							
	REP							
	WT							
	REP							
	WT							
	REP							
	WT							
	REP							
	WT							
	REP							
	WT							
	REP							
	WT							
	REP							
	WT							

STRETCHING   Time Spent: _____

EXERCISE	Duration	Comments

Day of Week: M - T - W - Th - F - Sa - Su
Date: _____

NUTRITION LOG

DAILY GOAL	Calories	Protein (gr)	Carbs (gr)	Fat (gr)	Water (oz)	Comments

ACTUAL CONSUMPTION

FOODS	Calories	Protein (gr)	Carbs (gr)	Fat (gr)	Water (oz)	Comments
AM/PM MEAL ONE						
AM/PM MEAL TWO						
AM/PM MEAL THREE						
AM/PM MEAL FOUR						
AM/PM MEAL FIVE						
AM/PM MEAL SIX						
TOTAL						

SUPPLEMENTS

WORKOUT LOG

Day of Week: M - T - W - Th - F - Sa - Su

Date @ Time: _____

CARDIOVASCULAR WORKOUT   Time Spent: _____

EXERCISE	Time	Distance	Average HR or Intensity Level	Calories Burned	Comments

STRENGTH TRAINING   { ❏ Upper Body ❏ Lower Body ❏ Abs }   Time Spent: _____

EXERCISE		1st Set	2nd Set	3rd Set	4th Set	5th Set	6th Set	Comments
	REP							
	WT							
	REP							
	WT							
	REP							
	WT							
	REP							
	WT							
	REP							
	WT							
	REP							
	WT							
	REP							
	WT							
	REP							
	WT							

STRETCHING   Time Spent: _____

EXERCISE	Duration	Comments

Day of Week: M - T - W - Th - F - Sa - Su
Date: _____

NUTRITION LOG

DAILY GOAL	Calories	Protein (gr)	Carbs (gr)	Fat (gr)	Water (oz)	Comments

ACTUAL CONSUMPTION

FOODS	Calories	Protein (gr)	Carbs (gr)	Fat (gr)	Water (oz)	Comments
AM PM **MEAL ONE**						
AM PM **MEAL TWO**						
AM PM **MEAL THREE**						
AM PM **MEAL FOUR**						
AM PM **MEAL FIVE**						
AM PM **MEAL SIX**						
TOTAL						

SUPPLEMENTS

_____

_____

WORKOUT LOG

Day of Week: M - T - W - Th - F - Sa - Su
Date @ Time: _____

CARDIOVASCULAR WORKOUT   Time Spent: _____

EXERCISE	Time	Distance	Average HR or Intensity Level	Calories Burned	Comments

STRENGTH TRAINING { ❏ Upper Body ❏ Lower Body ❏ Abs } Time Spent: _____

EXERCISE		1st Set	2nd Set	3rd Set	4th Set	5th Set	6th Set	Comments
	REP							
	WT							
	REP							
	WT							
	REP							
	WT							
	REP							
	WT							
	REP							
	WT							
	REP							
	WT							
	REP							
	WT							
	REP							
	WT							

STRETCHING   Time Spent: _____

EXERCISE	Duration	Comments

Day of Week: M - T - W - Th - F - Sa - Su
Date: _____

NUTRITION LOG

DAILY GOAL	Calories	Protein (gr)	Carbs (gr)	Fat (gr)	Water (oz)	Comments

ACTUAL CONSUMPTION

FOODS	Calories	Protein (gr)	Carbs (gr)	Fat (gr)	Water (oz)	Comments
AM PM MEAL ONE						
AM PM MEAL TWO						
AM PM MEAL THREE						
AM PM MEAL FOUR						
AM PM MEAL FIVE						
AM PM MEAL SIX						
TOTAL						

SUPPLEMENTS

WORKOUT LOG

Day of Week: M - T - W - Th - F - Sa - Su
Date @ Time: _____

CARDIOVASCULAR WORKOUT   Time Spent: _____

EXERCISE	Time	Distance	Average HR or Intensity Level	Calories Burned	Comments

STRENGTH TRAINING   { ☐ Upper Body ☐ Lower Body ☐ Abs }   Time Spent: _____

EXERCISE		1st Set	2nd Set	3rd Set	4th Set	5th Set	6th Set	Comments
	REP							
	WT							
	REP							
	WT							
	REP							
	WT							
	REP							
	WT							
	REP							
	WT							
	REP							
	WT							
	REP							
	WT							
	REP							
	WT							

STRETCHING   Time Spent: _____

EXERCISE	Duration	Comments

Day of Week: M - T - W - Th - F - Sa - Su

Date: _____

NUTRITION LOG

DAILY GOAL	Calories	Protein (gr)	Carbs (gr)	Fat (gr)	Water (oz)	Comments

ACTUAL CONSUMPTION

FOODS	Calories	Protein (gr)	Carbs (gr)	Fat (gr)	Water (oz)	Comments
AM PM MEAL ONE						
AM PM MEAL TWO						
AM PM MEAL THREE						
AM PM MEAL FOUR						
AM PM MEAL FIVE						
AM PM MEAL SIX						
TOTAL						

SUPPLEMENTS

_____

_____

WORKOUT LOG

Day of Week: M - T - W - Th - F - Sa - Su
Date @ Time: _____

CARDIOVASCULAR WORKOUT   Time Spent: _____

EXERCISE	Time	Distance	Average HR or Intensity Level	Calories Burned	Comments

STRENGTH TRAINING   { ☐ Upper Body ☐ Lower Body ☐ Abs } Time Spent: _____

EXERCISE		1st Set	2nd Set	3rd Set	4th Set	5th Set	6th Set	Comments
	REP							
	WT							
	REP							
	WT							
	REP							
	WT							
	REP							
	WT							
	REP							
	WT							
	REP							
	WT							
	REP							
	WT							
	REP							
	WT							

STRETCHING   Time Spent: _____

EXERCISE	Duration	Comments

Day of Week: M - T - W - Th - F - Sa - Su
Date: _____

NUTRITION LOG

DAILY GOAL	Calories	Protein (gr)	Carbs (gr)	Fat (gr)	Water (oz)	Comments

ACTUAL CONSUMPTION

FOODS	Calories	Protein (gr)	Carbs (gr)	Fat (gr)	Water (oz)	Comments
MEAL ONE AM/PM						
MEAL TWO AM/PM						
MEAL THREE AM/PM						
MEAL FOUR AM/PM						
MEAL FIVE AM/PM						
MEAL SIX AM/PM						
TOTAL						

SUPPLEMENTS

listen|imagine|view|experience

AUDIO BOOK DOWNLOAD INCLUDED WITH THIS BOOK!

In your hands you hold a complete digital entertainment package. Besides purchasing the paper version of this book, this book includes a free download of the audio version of this book. Simply use the code listed below when visiting our website. Once downloaded to your computer, you can listen to the book through your computer's speakers, burn it to an audio CD or save the file to your portable music device (such as Apple's popular iPod) and listen on the go!

How to get your free audio book digital download:

1. Visit www.tatepublishing.com and click on the e|LIVE logo on the home page.
2. Enter the following coupon code:
   43df-d460-15a0-599d-a217-4d29-9a4c-26a4
3. Download the audio book from your e|LIVE digital locker and begin enjoying your new digital entertainment package today!